STUDENT LABORATORY MANUAL

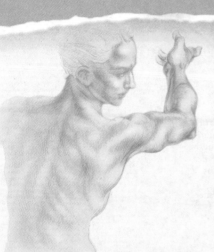

CAROLYN JARVIS, PhD, APN, CNP

Professor of Nursing
School of Nursing
Illinois Wesleyan University
Bloomington, Illinois
and
Family Nurse Practitioner
Bloomington, Illinois

Physical Examination & Health Assessment

6th Edition

ELSEVIER
SAUNDERS

3251 Riverport Lane
St. Louis, Missouri 63043

STUDENT LABORATORY MANUAL FOR PHYSICAL EXAMINATION AND   978-1-4377-1445-6
HEALTH ASSESSMENT

ISBN: 978-1-4377-1445-6

Executive Editor: Robin Carter
Developmental Editor: Deanna Dedeke
Publishing Services Manager: Deborah L. Vogel
Senior Project Manager: Jodi M. Willard
Design Direction: Teresa McBryan

Printed in the United States of America

Last digit is the print number: 9   8   7   6   5   4   3   2

CONTRIBUTORS

Carla Graf, MS, RN, CNS-BC
Geriatric Clinical Nurse Specialist
University of California San Francisco;
Assistant Clinical Professor
UCSF School of Nursing
San Francisco, California
*Chapter 30: Functional Assessment of
the Older Adult*

Joyce K. Keithley, DNSc, RN, FAAN
Professor
Department of Adult Health Nursing
Rush University College of Nursing
Rush University Medical Center
Chicago, Illinois
Chapter 11: Nutritional Assessment

Melissa A. Lee, MS, RN, CNS-BC
Medical-Surgical Clinical Nurse Specialist
University of California San Francisco
  Medical Center
San Francisco, California
*Chapter 30: Functional Assessment of
the Older Adult*

Rachel E. Spector, PhD, RN, CTN, FAAN
Cultural Care Consultant
Needham, Massachusetts
Chapter 2: Cultural Competence: Cultural Care

Deborah E. Swenson, MSN, ARNP, C-WHCNP
Women's Health Care Nurse Practitioner
Perinatal Medicine Clinic
Swedish Medical Center
OBSTETRIX Medical Group
Seattle, Washington
Chapter 29: The Pregnant Woman

Sharon R. Redding, MN, RN, CNE
Nurse Educator
Alegent Bergan Mercy Medical Center
Omaha, Nebraska
Chapters 1-26, 29-30: New Review Questions

PREFACE

This *Student Laboratory Manual* is intended for you, the student, as a study guide and laboratory manual to accompany the textbook *Physical Examination & Health Assessment*, 6th edition. You will use it in two places: in your own study area and in the skills laboratory.

As a study guide, this workbook highlights and reinforces the content from the text. Each chapter corresponds to a chapter in the textbook and contains exercises and questions in varying formats to provide the repetition needed to synthesize and master content from the text. Fill out the lab manual chapter and answer the questions before coming to the skills laboratory. This will reinforce your lectures, expose any areas in which you have questions for your clinical instructor, and prime you for the skills laboratory/clinical experience.

Once in the skills laboratory, use the *Student Laboratory Manual* as a direct clinical tool. Each chapter contains assessment forms on perforated, tear-out pages. Usually you will work in pairs and perform the regional physical examinations on each other under the tutelage of your instructor. As you perform the examination on your peer, you can fill out the write-up sheet and assessment form to be handed in and checked by the instructor.

Chapter 6, Substance Use Assessment, has been added to the manual to accompany new material in the 6th edition textbook.

FEATURES

Each chapter is divided into two parts—cognitive and clinical—and contains:
- Purpose—a brief summary of the material you are learning in the chapter.
- Reading Assignment—the corresponding chapter and page numbers from the *Physical Examination & Health Assessment* textbook, as well as space for your instructor to assign journal articles.
- Media Assignment—the corresponding video assignment from the Physical Examination and Health Assessment DVD Series, which is adapted from the *Physical Examination & Health Assessment* textbook, as well as space for your instructor to assign relevant audio or online learning modules.
- Glossary—important or specialized terms from the textbook chapter with accompanying definitions.
- Study Guide—specific short-answer and fill-in questions to help you highlight and learn content from the chapter. Critical thinking questions from the video assessment series are included to coordinate the reading and video assignments. Important illustrations of human anatomy have been reproduced from the textbook with the labels deleted so you can identify and fill in the names of the structures yourself.
- Review Questions—new and revised multiple-choice questions, matching, and short-answer questions so you can monitor your own mastery of the material. Take the self-exam when you are ready and then check your answers against the answer key provided in Appendix A.
- Clinical Objectives—behavioral objectives that you should achieve during your peer practice in the regional examinations.
- Regional Write-Up Sheets—complete yet succinct physical exam forms that you can use in the skills lab or in the clinical setting. These serve as a memory prompt, listing key history questions and physical examination steps, and as a means of recording data during the patient encounter.
- Narrative Summary Forms—SOAP format, so you can learn to chart narrative accounts of the history and physical exam findings. These forms have accompanying sketches of regional anatomy and are especially useful for those studying advanced practice roles.

Learning the skills of history taking and physical examination requires two types of practice: cognitive and clinical. It is my hope that this manual will help you achieve both of these learning and practice modalities.

CAROLYN JARVIS

ACKNOWLEDGMENTS

I am grateful to those on the team at Elsevier who worked on the *Student Laboratory Manual*. My thanks extend to Robin Carter, Executive Editor, for her leadership, encouragement, and organizational support; to Deanna Dedeke, Developmental Editor, and Kevin Korinek, Editorial Assistant, for their extreme helpfulness and for their guidance and coordination in various stages of production; and to Jodi Willard, Senior Project Manager, for her support and organization during production.

CONTENTS

UNIT 1: ASSESSMENT OF THE WHOLE PERSON

UNIT 2: APPROACH TO THE CLINICAL SETTING

UNIT 3: PHYSICAL EXAMINATION

UNIT 4: INTEGRATION OF THE HEALTH SYSTEM

APPENDIXES

CHAPTER 1

Evidence-Based Assessment

PURPOSE

This chapter discusses the characteristics of evidence-based practice, diagnostic reasoning, the nursing process, and critical thinking. This chapter also introduces the concept of health, helps you understand that it is the definition of health that determines the kinds of factors that are assessed, and shows you that the amount of data gathered during assessment varies with the person's age, developmental state, physical condition, risk factors, and culture.

READING ASSIGNMENT

Jarvis: *Physical Examination and Health Assessment*, 6th ed., Chapter 1, pp. 1-10.

GLOSSARY

Study the following terms after completing the reading assignment. You should be able to cover the definition on the right and define the term out loud.

Assessment . . . . the collection of data about an individual's health state

Biomedical model . . . . the Western European/North American tradition that views health as the absence of disease

Complete database . . . . a complete health history and full physical examination

Critical thinking . . . . simultaneously problem-solving while self-improving one's own thinking ability

Diagnostic reasoning . . . . a method of collecting and analyzing clinical information with the following components: (1) attending to initially available cues, (2) formulating diagnostic hypotheses, (3) gathering data relative to the tentative hypotheses, (4) evaluating each hypothesis with the new data collected, and (5) arriving at a final diagnosis

Emergency database . . . . rapid collection of the database, often compiled concurrently with lifesaving measures

Environment. . . . . the total of all the conditions and elements that make up the surroundings and influence the development of a person

Evidence-based practice. . . . . . a systematic approach emphasizing the best research evidence, the clinician's experience, patient preferences and values, physical examination, and assessment

Focused database. . . . . one used for a limited or short-term problem; concerns mainly one problem, one cue complex, or one body system

Follow-up database. . . . . used in all settings to monitor progress on short-term or chronic health problems

Holistic health . . . . the view that the mind, body, and spirit are interdependent and function as a whole within the environment

Medical diagnosis . . . . used to evaluate the cause and etiology of disease; focus is on the function or malfunction of a specific organ system

Nursing diagnosis . . . . used to evaluate the response of the whole person to actual or potential health problems

Nursing process . . . . a method of collecting and analyzing clinical information with the following components: (1) assessment, (2) diagnosis, (3) outcome identification, (4) planning, (5) implementation, and (6) evaluation

Objective data . . . . what the health professional observes by inspecting, palpating, percussing, and auscultating during the physical examination

Prevention . . . . any action directed toward promoting health and preventing the occurrence of disease

Subjective data. . . . . what the person says about himself or herself during history taking

Wellness. . . . . a dynamic process and view of health; a move toward optimal functioning

STUDY GUIDE

After completing the reading assignment, you should be able to answer the following questions in the spaces provided.

1. The steps of the diagnostic reasoning process are listed below. Consider the clinical example given for "cue recognition," and fill in the remaining diagnostic reasoning steps.

Stage	Example
Cue recognition	A.J., 62-year-old male, appears pale, diaphoretic, and anxious
Hypothesis formulation	
Data gathering for hypothesis testing	
Hypothesis evaluation	

2. One of the critical-thinking skills is identifying assumptions. Explain how the following statement contains an assumption. How would you get the facts in this situation? *"Ellen, you have to break up with your boyfriend. He is too rough with you. He is no good for you."*

3. Another critical-thinking skill involves validation, or checking the accuracy and reliability of data. Describe how you would validate the following data.

   Mr. Quinn tells you his weight this morning on the clinic scale was 165 lbs.

   The primary counselor tells you Ellen is depressed and angry about being admitted to residential treatment in the clinic.

   When auscultating the heart, you hear a blowing, swooshing sound between the first and second heart sounds.

4. List the barriers to evidence-based practice, both on an individual level and on an organizational level.

5. Differentiate **subjective** data from **objective** data by placing an **S** or an **O** after each of the following: complaint of sore shoulder _____; unconscious _____; blood in the urine _____; family has just moved to a new area _____; dizziness _____; sore throat _____; earache _____; weight gain _____.

6. How are medical diagnosis and nursing diagnosis similar?

   How are they different?

7. For the following situations, state the type of data collection you would perform (i.e., *complete* database, *focused* or problem-centered database, *follow-up* database, *emergency* database).

    Barbiturate overdose _____; ambulatory, apparently well individual who presents at outpatient clinic with a rash _____; first visit to a health care provider for a "checkup" _____; recently placed on antihypertensive medication _____.

8. Discuss the impact that racial and cultural diversity of individuals has on the U.S. health care system.

9. List three health care interactions you have experienced yourself with another person from a culture or ethnicity different from your own. You may have been the patient or the provider—it makes no difference.

10. Using one sentence or group of phrases, how would you describe your own health state to someone you are meeting for the first time?

REVIEW QUESTIONS

This test is for you to check your own mastery of the content. Answers are provided in Appendix A.

1. The concept of health has expanded in the past 40 years. Select the phrase that reflects the most narrow description of health.

   a. the absence of disease
   b. a dynamic process toward optimal functioning
   c. depends on an interaction of mind, body, and spirit within the environment
   d. prevention of disease

2. Select the most complete description of a database.

   a. subjective and objective data gathered by a health practitioner from a patient
   b. objective data obtained from a patient through inspection, percussion, palpation, and auscultation
   c. a summary of a patient's record, including laboratory studies
   d. subjective and objective data gathered from a patient plus the results of any diagnostic studies completed

3. Nursing diagnoses, based on assessment of a number of factors, give nurses a common language with which to communicate nursing findings. The best description of a nursing diagnosis is:

   a. used to evaluate the etiology of a disease.
   b. a pattern of coping.
   c. a concise description of actual or potential health problems or of wellness strengths.
   d. the patient's perception of and satisfaction with his or her own health status.

4. Depending on the clinical situation, the nurse may establish one of four kinds of database. A focused database is described as:

   a. including a complete health history and full physical examination.
   b. concerning mainly one problem.
   c. evaluation of a previously identified problem.
   d. rapid collection of data in conjunction with lifesaving measures.

5. Individuals should be seen at regular intervals for health care. The frequency of these visits:

   a. is most efficient if performed on an annual basis.
   b. is not important. There is no recommendation for the frequency of health care.
   c. varies, depending on the person's illness and wellness needs.
   d. is based on the practitioner's clinical experience.

6. Cultural diversity is currently considered when discussing health assessment and care. From a nursing perspective, the most accurate description of this phenomenon is:

   a. nursing is inherently a transcultural phenomenon. The process of helping people involves at least two people having different cultural orientations.
   b. a consideration when the nurse is caring for someone identified as a minority among the local population.
   c. the consideration of the needs of the population of the United States that does not have European ancestry.
   d. an area that has always been of consideration to nursing and is included in most nursing curricula.

7. Evidence-based nursing practice can be described as:

   a. combining clinical expertise with the use of nursing research to provide the best care for patients while considering the patient's values and circumstances.
   b. appraising and looking at the implications of one or two articles as they relate to the culture and ethnicity of the patient.
   c. completing a literature search to find relevant articles that utilize nursing research so as to encourage nurses to use good practices.
   d. finding value-based resources to justify nursing actions when working with patients of diverse cultural backgrounds.

8. What can be determined when the nurse clusters data as part of the critical-thinking process?

   a. This identifies problems that may be urgent and require immediate action by the nurse.
   b. This step of the process involves recognizing inconsistencies in the data.
   c. The nurse recognizes patterns and relationships among the data.
   d. Risk factors can be determined so the nurse knows how to offer health teaching.

NOTES

Cultural Competence: Cultural Care

PURPOSE

This chapter discusses the demographic profile of the United States, the National Standards for Culturally and Linguistically Appropriate Services in Health Care, the composition of heritage and the process of heritage assessment, traditional HEALTH/ILLNESS beliefs and practices, and the steps to cultural competency. At the end of the chapter, you will have increased your knowledge of and sensitivity to the cultural dimensions of HEALTH care, be able to perform a heritage assessment, and determine HEALTH/ILLNESS beliefs and practices.

READING ASSIGNMENT

Jarvis: *Physical Examination and Health Assessment*, 6th ed., Chapter 2, pp. 11-28.

GLOSSARY

Study the following terms after completing the reading assignment. You should be able to cover the definition on the right and define the term out loud.

Cultural and linguistic competence . . . . a set of congruent behaviors, attitudes, and policies that come together in a system among professionals that enables work in cross-cultural situations

Cultural care nursing . . . . professional health care that is culturally sensitive, appropriate, and competent

Culture . . . . the nonphysical attributes of a person—the thoughts, communications, actions, beliefs, values, and institutions of racial, ethnic, religious, or social groups

Culture-bound syndrome . . . . a condition that is culturally defined

Ethnicity . . . . a social group within the social system that claims to possess variable traits such as a common geographic origin, migratory status, and religion

Ethnocentrism . . . . tendency to view your own way of life as the most desirable, acceptable, or best and to act superior to another culture's lifeways

Folk healer . . . . lay healer in the person's culture apart from the biomedical/scientific health care system

Health/illness . . . . the balance/imbalance of the person, both within one's being (physical, mental, and/or spiritual) and in the outside world (natural, communal, and/or metaphysical)

Heritage consistency . . . . the degree to which a person's lifestyle reflects his or her traditional heritage, whether it is American Indian, European, Asian, African, or Hispanic

Religion . . . . the belief in a divine or superhuman power or powers to be obeyed and worshiped as the creator(s) and ruler(s) of the universe; and a system of beliefs, practices, and ethical values

Socialization . . . . the process of being raised within a culture and acquiring the characteristics of that group

Title VI of the Civil
Rights Act of 1964 . . . . a federal law that mandates that when people with limited English proficiency (LEP) seek health care in health care settings such as hospitals, nursing homes, clinics, daycare centers, and mental health centers, services cannot be denied to them

Values . . . . a desirable or undesirable state of affairs and a universal feature of all cultures

STUDY GUIDE

After completing the reading assignment, you should be able to answer the following questions in the spaces provided.

1. Describe the provisions of Title VI of the Civil Rights Act of 1964.

2. Describe the rationale and components of cultural care nursing.

3. Differentiate the norms of a traditional heritage and those of a modern heritage.

4. List the 4 basic characteristics of culture.

5. List 4 examples of health practices that may be promoted by a given patient's religious beliefs.

6. List and describe 3 factors related to socialization.

7. List and define 3 major theories on the ways in which people view the causes of illness.

8. Define the *yin/yang theory* of health and illness, and relate this to different types of foods.

9. Define the *hot/cold theory* of health and illness, and relate this to different types of foods and illnesses.

10. List at least 5 names for various folk healers and the culture they represent.

11. Define the term *culture-bound syndrome,* and give some examples from the African-American, Hispanic, American Indian, and European-American cultures.

12. Describe 5 methods of complementary interventions.

REVIEW QUESTIONS

This test is for you to check your own mastery of the content. Answers are provided in Appendix A.

1. Religion is best described as:

   a. an organized system of beliefs concerning the cause, nature, and purpose of the universe.
   b. belief in a divine or superhuman spirit to be obeyed and worshiped.
   c. affiliation with one of the 1200 recognized religions in the United States.
   d. the following of established rituals, especially in conjunction with health-seeking behaviors.

2. The major factor contributing to the need for cultural care nursing is:

   a. an increasing birth rate.
   b. limited access to health care services.
   c. demographic change.
   d. a decreasing rate of immigration.

3. "Culturally competent" implies that the nurse:

   a. is prepared in nursing.
   b. possesses knowledge of the traditions of diverse peoples.
   c. applies underlying knowledge to providing nursing care.
   d. understands the cultural context of the patient's situation.

4. Many of the traditional definitions of HEALTH tend to focus on:

   a. beliefs of body and mind.
   b. equilibrium with others.
   c. physical, mental, and spiritual harmony.
   d. ability to perform activities of daily living.

5. ILLNESS may be described as an imbalance of hot and cold among people of:

   a. Asian-American heritage.
   b. African-American heritage.
   c. Hispanic-American heritage.
   d. American Indian heritage.

6. An amulet may be used to protect a person from:

   a. the evil eye.
   b. being kidnapped.
   c. exposure to bacterial infections.
   d. an unexpected fall.

7. The term "empacho," which is used in the Hispanic culture, can be explained as:

   a. a folk healer who specializes in the use of herbs and tonics.
   b. an example of a culture-bound syndrome that has no equivalent from a biomedical/scientific perspective.
   c. a self-care complementary intervention.
   d. a reward for good behavior.

8. The first step to cultural competency by a nurse is to:

   a. identify the meaning of health to the patient.
   b. understand how a health care delivery system works.
   c. develop a frame of reference as to traditional health care practices.
   d. understand your own heritage and its basis in cultural values.

SKILLS LABORATORY/CLINICAL SETTING

You are now ready for the clinical component of this chapter. The purpose of the clinical component is to collect data for a heritage assessment on a peer in the skills laboratory or on a patient in the clinical setting. Although you may not have been assigned chapters on the health history as yet, the questions in the heritage assessment tool are clearly defined and should pose no problem. The best experience would be for you to pair up with a peer from a cultural heritage *different* from your own. If this is not possible, you still will gain insight and sensitivity into the cultural dimensions of health and will gain mastery of the assessment tool.

BOX 2-1   HERITAGE ASSESSMENT

1. Where were you born? _____

2. Where were your parents/grandparents born?

   a. Mother: _____
   b. Father: _____
   c. Mother's mother: _____
   d. Mother's father: _____
   e. Father's mother: _____
   f. Father's father: _____

3. How many brothers _____ and sisters _____ do you have?

4. In what setting did you grow up? Urban _____ Rural _____ Suburban _____

   Where? _____

5. In what country did your parents/grandparents grow up?

   a. Mother: _____
   b. Father: _____
   c. Mother's mother: _____
   d. Mother's father: _____
   e. Father's mother: _____
   f. Father's father: _____

6. How old were you when you came to the United States? _____

7. How old were your parents/grandparents when they came to the United States?

   a. Mother: _____
   b. Father: _____
   c. Mother's mother: _____
   d. Mother's father: _____
   e. Father's mother: _____
   f. Father's father: _____

8. When you were growing up, who lived with you? _____

9. Have you maintained contact with:

   a. Aunts, uncles, cousins? _____ Yes _____ No
   b. Brothers and sisters? _____ Yes _____ No
   c. Parents? _____ Yes _____ No
   d. Grandparents? _____ Yes _____ No

10. Does most of your family live near you? _____ Yes _____ No

11. Approximately how often did you visit your family members who lived outside your home?

    _____ Daily _____ Weekly _____ Monthly _____ Less than once a year _____ Never

12. Was your original family name changed? _____ Yes _____ No

13. What is your religious preference? _____ Catholic _____ Jewish

    _____ Protestant (denomination): _____ Other _____ None

14. Is your significant other of the same religion? _____ Yes _____ No

15. Is your significant other of the same ethnic background as you? _____ Yes _____ No

16. What kind of school did you attend? _____ Public _____ Private _____ Parochial

17. As an adult, do you live in a neighborhood where the neighbors are the same religion and ethnic background as yourself? _____ Yes _____ No

18. Do you belong to a religious institution? _____ Yes _____ No

19. Would you describe yourself as an active member? _____ Yes _____ No

20. How often do you attend your religious institution? _____ More than once a week _____ Weekly _____ Monthly _____ Special holidays only _____ Never

21. Do you practice your religion or other spiritual practices in your home? _____ Yes _____ No

    If yes, please specify: _____ Praying _____ Bible reading _____ Diet

    _____ Celebrating religious holidays _____ Meditating

    Other: _____

22. Do you prepare foods of your ethnic background? _____ Yes _____ No

23. Do you participate in ethnic activities? _____ Yes _____ No

    If yes, specify: _____ Singing _____ Holiday celebrations _____ Dancing

    _____ Costumes _____ Festivals _____ Other

24. Are your friends from the same religious background? _____ Yes _____ No

25. Are your friends of the same ethnic background as you? _____ Yes _____ No

26. What is your native (non-English) language? _____

    Do you speak this language? _____ Prefer _____ Occasionally _____ Rarely

27. Do you read in your native language? _____ Prefer _____ Occasionally _____ Rarely

(You may score this assessment by giving 1 point to each positive answer from the yes/no questions 9 through 27. The exception: if a person's name was not changed, then he or she gets the point. The higher the score, the more likely the person is to use health practices relevant to his or her traditional heritage.)

From Spector, R.E. (2009). *Cultural diversity in health and illness* (7th ed., pp. 365-367). Upper Saddle River, NJ: Prentice Hall.

HEALTH AND ILLNESS BELIEFS AND PRACTICES DETERMINATION

The next set of questions relates to *your own* personal health and illness beliefs and practices.

1. How do you define health?

2. How do you rate your health? *(circle 1)*
    a.   Excellent
    b.   Good
    c.   Fair
    d.   Poor

3. How do you describe illness?

4. What do you believe causes illness? *(circle all that apply)*
    a.   Environmental change
    b.   Evil eye
    c.   Exposure to drafts
    d.   God's punishment
    e.   Grief and loss
    f.   Hexes and spells
    g.   Incorrect food combinations
    h.   Not enough work
    i.   Overwork
    j.   Poor eating habits
    k.   Viruses, bacteria
    l.   Witchcraft
    m.   Other

5. What did your mother do to maintain and protect your health?

6. How do you maintain and protect your health?

7. What home remedies did your mother use to restore your health?

8. What home remedies do you use?

9. Healing and curing are the same. _____ Yes _____ No

10. What do you believe brings healing?

NOTES

PURPOSE

This chapter discusses the process of communication; presents the techniques of interviewing including open-ended versus closed questions, the 9 types of examiner responses, the 10 "traps" of interviewing, and nonverbal skills; and considers variations in technique that are necessary for individuals of different ages, for those with special needs, and for culturally diverse people.

READING ASSIGNMENT

Jarvis: *Physical Examination and Health Assessment*, 6th ed., Chapter 3, pp. 29-48.

GLOSSARY

Study the following terms after completing the reading assignment. You should be able to cover the definition on the right and define the term out loud.

Ad hoc interpreter . . . . using a patient's family member, friend, or child as interpreter for a limited English proficiency (LEP) patient

Animism . . . . imagining that inanimate objects (e.g., a blood pressure cuff) come alive and have human characteristics

Avoidance language . . . . the use of euphemisms to avoid reality or to hide feelings

Clarification . . . . examiner's response used when the patient's word choice is ambiguous or confusing

Closed questions . . . . questions that ask for specific information; elicit a short, one- or two-word answer, a "yes" or "no," or a forced choice

Confrontation . . . . response in which examiner gives honest feedback about what he or she has seen or felt after observing a certain patient action, feeling, or statement

Distancing . . . . the use of impersonal speech to put space between the self and a threat

Elderspeak . . . . infantilizing and demeaning language used by a health professional when speaking to an older adult

Electronic health recording. . . direct computer entry of the patient health record while in the patient's presence

Empathy . . . . viewing the world from the other person's inner frame of reference while remaining yourself; recognizing and accepting the other person's feelings without criticism

Ethnocentrism . . . . the tendency to view your own way of life as the most desirable, acceptable, or best and to act in a superior manner to another culture's lifeways

Explanation . . . . examiner's statements that inform the patient; examiner shares factual and objective information

Facilitation . . . . examiner's response that encourages the patient to say more, to continue with the story

Geographic privacy. . . . . private room or space with only examiner and patient present

Interpretation . . . . examiner's statement that is not based on direct observation, but is based on examiner's inference or conclusion; it links events, makes associations, or implies cause

Interview. . . . . meeting between examiner and patient with the goal of gathering a complete health history

Jargon . . . . using medical vocabulary with patient in an exclusionary and paternalistic way

Leading question. . . . . a question that implies that one answer would be better than another

Nonverbal communication . . . message conveyed through body language—posture, gestures, facial expression, eye contact, touch, and even where one places the chairs

Open-ended question . . . . asks for longer narrative information; unbiased; leaves the person free to answer in any way

Reflection . . . . examiner response that echoes the patient's words; repeats part of what patient has just said

Summary. . . . . final review of what examiner understands patient has said; condenses facts and presents a survey of how the examiner perceives the health problem or need

Telegraphic speech . . . . speech used by age 3 or 4 in which three- or four-word sentences contain only the essential words

Verbal communication . . . . . . messages sent through spoken words, vocalizations, tone of voice

Jarvis, Carolyn: PHYSICAL EXAMINATION AND HEALTH ASSESSMENT: Sixth Edition,
Student Laboratory Manual. Copyright © 2012, 2008, 2004, 2000, 1996 by Saunders, an imprint of Elsevier Inc. All rights reserved.

STUDY GUIDE

After completing the reading assignment, you should be able to answer the following questions in the spaces provided.

1. List 8 items of information that should be communicated to the patient concerning the terms or expectations of the interview.

2. Describe the points to consider in preparing the physical setting for the interview.

3. List the pros and cons of note-taking during the interview.

4. Contrast open-ended versus closed questions, and explain the purpose of each during the interview.

5. List the 9 types of examiner responses that could be used during the interview, and give a short example of each.

6. List the 10 traps of interviewing, and give a short example of each.

7. State at least 7 types of nonverbal behaviors that an interviewer could make.

8. State a useful phrase to use as a closing when ending the interview.

9. Discuss special considerations when interviewing the older adult.

10. Discuss ways you would modify your interviewing technique when working with a hearing-impaired person.

11. Formulate a response you would make to a patient who has spoken to you in ways you interpret as sexually aggressive.

12. Discuss the ways that nonverbal behavior may vary cross-culturally.

13. List at least 5 points to consider when using an interpreter during an interview.

REVIEW QUESTIONS

This test is for you to check your own mastery of the content. Answers are provided in Appendix A.

1. The practitioner, entering the examining room to meet a patient for the first time, states: "Hello, I'm M.M., and I'm here to gather some information from you and to perform your examination. This will take about 30 minutes. D.D. is a student working with me. If it's all right with you, she will remain during the examination." Which of the following must be added in order to cover all aspects of the interview contract?

   a. a statement regarding confidentiality, patient costs, and the expectation of each person
   b. the purpose of the interview and the role of the examiner
   c. time and place of the interview and a confidentiality statement
   d. an explicit purpose of the interview and a description of the physical examination, including diagnostic studies

2. An accurate understanding of the other person's feelings within a communication context is an example of:

   a. empathy.
   b. liking others.
   c. facilitation.
   d. a nonverbal listening technique.

3. You have come into a patient's room to conduct an admission interview. Because you are expecting a phone call, you stand near the door during the interview. A more appropriate approach would be to:

   a. arrange to have someone page you so you can sit on the side of the bed.
   b. have someone else answer the phone so you can sit facing the patient.
   c. use this approach given the circumstances; it is correct.
   d. arrange for a time free of interruptions after the initial physical examination is complete.

4. Students frequently ask teachers, "May I ask you a question?" This is an example of:

   a. an open-ended question.
   b. a reflective question.
   c. a closed question.
   d. a double-barreled question.

5. During a patient interview, you recognize the need to use interpretation. This verbal response:

   a. is the same as clarification.
   b. is a summary of a statement made by a patient.
   c. is used to focus on a particular aspect of what the patient has just said.
   d. is based on the interviewer's inference from the data that have been presented.

6. A good rule for an interviewer is to:

   a. stop the patient each time something is said that is not understood.
   b. spend more time listening to the patient than talking.
   c. consistently think of your next response so the patient will know you understand him.
   d. use "why" questions to seek clarification of unusual symptoms or behavior.

7. During an interview, a patient denies having any anxiety. The patient frequently changes position in the chair, holds his arms folded tight against his chest, and has little eye contact with the interviewer. The interviewer should:

   a. use confrontation to bring the discrepancy between verbal and nonverbal behavior to the patient's attention.
   b. proceed with the interview. Patients usually are truthful with a health care practitioner.
   c. make a mental note to discuss the behavior after the physical examination is completed.
   d. proceed with the interview and examination as outlined on the agency assessment form. The patient's behavior is appropriate for the circumstances.

8. Touch should be used during the interview:

   a. only with individuals from a Western culture.
   b. as a routine way of establishing contact with the person and communicating empathy.
   c. only with patients of the same gender.
   d. only if the interviewer knows the person well.

9. Children are usually brought for health care by a parent. At about what age should the interviewer begin to question the child himself or herself regarding presenting symptoms?

   a. 5 years
   b. 7 years
   c. 9 years
   d. 11 years

10. Because of adolescents' developmental level, not all interviewing techniques can be used with them. The two to be avoided are:

   a. facilitation and clarification.
   b. confrontation and explanation.
   c. empathy and interpretations.
   d. silence and reflection.

11. Knowledge of the use of personal space is helpful for the health care provider. Personal distance is generally considered to be:

   a. 0 to 1½ feet.
   b. 1½ to 4 feet.
   c. 4 to 12 feet.
   d. 12 or more feet.

12. Mr. B. tells you, "Everyone here ignores me." You respond, "Ignores you?" This technique is best described as:

   a. clarification.
   b. selective listening.
   c. reflecting.
   d. validation.

13. Active listening skills include all of the following except:

   a. taking detailed notes during the interview.
   b. watching for clues in body language.
   c. repeating statements back to the person to make sure you have understood.
   d. asking open-ended questions to explore the person's perspective.
   e. exploring the person's fears about his or her illness.

14. When interviewing patients who do not speak English or have limited proficiency, the examiner should:

    a. take advantage of family members who are readily available and willing to assist.
    b. use a qualified medical interpreter who is culturally literate.
    c. seek as much information as possible and then continue with the physical examination.
    d. wait until a qualified medical interpreter is available before starting the interview.

15. With older adults, what is the best approach to take with the interview?

    a. Proceed in a more organized and concise manner.
    b. Consider the fatigue of the aging person and break the interview into shorter segments.
    c. Ask a family member to complete some of the records while moving ahead with the interview.
    d. Raise your voice if the patient does not appear to hear you.

SKILLS LABORATORY/CLINICAL SETTING

Note that the clinical component of this chapter is the gathering of the complete health history. The history forms are included in Chapter 4.

NOTES

NOTES

The Complete Health History

PURPOSE

This chapter helps you learn the elements of a complete health history, interview a patient to gather the data for a complete health history, analyze the patient data, and record the history accurately.

READING ASSIGNMENT

Jarvis: *Physical Examination and Health Assessment,* 6th ed., Chapter 4, pp. 49–70.

STUDY GUIDE

After completing the reading assignment, you should be able to answer the following questions in the spaces provided.

1. State the purpose of the complete health history.

2. List and define the critical characteristics used to explore each symptom the patient identifies.

3. Define the elements of the health history: reason for seeking care; present health state or present illness; past history, family history; review of systems; functional patterns of living.

Jarvis, Carolyn: PHYSICAL EXAMINATION AND HEALTH ASSESSMENT: Sixth Edition,
Student Laboratory Manual. Copyright © 2012, 2008, 2004, 2000, 1996 by Saunders, an imprint of Elsevier Inc. All rights reserved.

4. Discuss the rationale for obtaining a family history.

5. Define a pedigree or genogram.

6. Discuss the rationale for obtaining a systems review.

7. Describe the items included in a functional assessment.

8. Describe the additions/modifications you would make in environment, pacing, and content when conducting a health history on an older adult.

REVIEW QUESTIONS

This test is for you to check your own mastery of the content. Answers are provided in Appendix A.

1. When reading a medical record, you see the following notation: Patient states, "I have had a cold for about a week, and now I am having difficulty breathing." This is an example of:

   a. past history.
   b. a review of systems.
   c. a functional assessment.
   d. a reason for seeking care.

2. You have reason to question the reliability of the information being provided by a patient. One way to verify the reliability within the context of the interview is to:

   a. rephrase the same questions later in the interview.
   b. review the patient's previous medical records.
   c. call the person identified as emergency contact to verify data provided.
   d. provide the patient with a printed history to complete and then compare the data provided.

3. The statement "Reason for seeking care" has replaced the "chief complaint." This change is significant because:

    a. "chief complaint" is really a diagnostic statement.
    b. the newer term allows another individual to supply the necessary information.
    c. the newer term incorporates wellness needs.
    d. "Reason for seeking care" can incorporate the history of present illness.

4. During an initial interview, the examiner says, "Mrs. J., tell me what you do when your headaches occur." With this question, the examiner is seeking information about:

    a. the patient's perception of the problem.
    b. aggravating or relieving factors.
    c. the frequency of the problem.
    d. the severity of the problem.

5. Which of the following is an appropriate recording of a patient's reason for seeking health care?

    a. angina pectoris, duration 2 hr
    b. substernal pain radiating to left axilla, 1 hr duration
    c. "grabbing" chest pain for 2 hr
    d. pleurisy, 2 days' duration

6. A genogram is useful in showing information concisely. It is used specifically for:

    a. past history.
    b. past health history, specifically hospitalizations.
    c. family history.
    d. the eight characteristics of presenting symptoms.

7. Select the best description of "review of systems" as part of the health history.

    a. the evaluation of the past and present health state of each body system
    b. a documentation of the problem as described by the patient
    c. the recording of the objective findings of the practitioner
    d. a statement that describes the overall health state of the patient

8. Which of the following is considered to be subjective?

    a. temperature of 101.2° F
    b. pulse rate of 96
    c. measured weight loss of 20 pounds since the previous measurement
    d. pain lasting 2 hours

9. When taking a health history for a child, what information, in addition to that for an adult, is usually obtained?

    a. coping and stress management
    b. a review of immunizations received
    c. environmental hazards
    d. hospitalization history

10. Functional assessment measures how a person manages day-to-day activities. The impact of a disease on the daily activities of older adults is referred to as:

    a. interpersonal relationship assessment.
    b. instrumental activities of daily living.
    c. reason for seeking care.
    d. disease burden.

11. The mnemonic *PQRSTU* is helpful for organizing the critical characteristics of a symptom. Give an example of a question that could be asked that relates to each of the letters.

P	
Q	
R	
S	
T	
U	

12. What two sections of the child's health history become separate sections because of their importance to current health status?

    a. play activities and rest patterns
    b. prenatal and postnatal status
    c. developmental and nutritional history
    d. accidents/injuries and immunizations

SKILLS LABORATORY/CLINICAL SETTING

You are now ready for the clinical component of the interview and health history chapters. The purpose of the clinical component is to practice conducting a complete health history on a peer in the skills laboratory and to achieve the following.

Clinical Objectives

1. Demonstrate knowledge of interviewing skills by arranging a private, quiet, comfortable setting; introducing yourself and stating your goals for the interview; posing open-ended and direct questions appropriately; listening to the patient in an attentive, nonjudgmental manner; choosing appropriate vocabulary that the patient understands.

2. Demonstrate knowledge of the components of a health history by recording the reason for seeking care in the person's own words; eliciting all the critical characteristics to describe the patient's symptom(s); gathering pertinent data for the past history, family history, and systems review; identifying self-care behaviors and risk factors from the functional assessment.

3. Record the history data accurately and as a reflection of what the patient believes the true health state to be.

Instructions

Work in pairs and obtain a complete health history from a peer. Although you already know each other as student colleagues, play your role straight as examiner or patient for the best learning experience. Be aware that some of the history questions cover personal content. When you are acting as the patient, you have the right to withhold an answer if you do not feel comfortable with the amount of material you will be asked to divulge. Your own rights to privacy must co-exist with the goals of the learning experience.

Familiarize yourself with the following history form and practice phrasing your questions ahead of time. Note that the language on this form is intended as a prompt for the examiner and must be translated into clear and appropriate phrases for the patient. As a beginning examiner, you will need to use one copy of the form as a worksheet during the actual interview and use a fresh copy of the form for your rewritten formal record.

WRITE-UP—HEALTH HISTORY

Date _____

Examiner _____

1. Biographical Data

Name _____ Phone _____

Address _____

Birth date _____ Birthplace _____

Age _____ Gender _____ Marital Status _____ Occupation _____

Race/ethnic origin _____ Employer _____

2. Source and Reliability

3. Reason for Seeking Care

4. Present Health or History of Present Illness

5. Past Health

Describe General Health _____

Childhood Illnesses _____

Accidents or Injuries (include age) _____

Serious or Chronic Illnesses (include age) _____

Hospitalizations (what for? location) _____

Operations (name procedure, age) _____

Obstetric History: Gravida _____ Term _____ Preterm _____

          (# Pregnancies)   (# Term pregnancies)   (# Preterm pregnancies)

                Ab/incomplete _____ Children living _____

                (# Abortions/Miscarriages)

Course of pregnancy _____

(Date delivery, length of pregnancy, length of labor, baby's weight and sex, vaginal delivery/cesarean section, complications, baby's condition)

Immunizations _____

Last examination date _____

Allergies _____ Reaction _____

Current medications _____

_____

6. Family History—Specify

Heart disease _____   Allergies _____
High blood pressure _____   Asthma _____
Stroke _____   Obesity _____
Diabetes _____   Alcoholism or drug addiction _____
Blood disorders _____   Mental illness _____
Breast/ovarian cancer _____   Suicide _____
Cancer (other) _____   Seizure disorder _____
Sickle cell _____   Kidney disease _____
Arthritis _____   Tuberculosis _____

Construct genogram below.

7. Review of Systems

(Circle both past health problems that have been resolved and current problems, including date of onset.)   (Describe circled items.)

General Overall Health State: Present weight (gain or loss, period of time, by diet or other factors), fatigue, weakness or malaise, fever, chills, sweats or night sweats.

Skin: History of skin disease (eczema, psoriasis, hives), pigment or color change, change in mole, excessive dryness or moisture, pruritus, excessive bruising, rash or lesion.

Hair: Recent loss, change in texture.

Nails: Change in shape, color, or brittleness.
   Health Promotion: Amount of sun exposure, method of self-care for skin and hair.

Head: Any unusually frequent or severe headache, any head injury, dizziness (syncope), or vertigo.

Eyes: Difficulty with vision (decreased acuity, blurring, blind spots), eye pain, diplopia (double vision), redness or swelling, watering or discharge, glaucoma or cataracts.
   Health Promotion: Wears glasses or contacts; last vision check or glaucoma test; how coping with loss of vision if any.

Ears: Earaches, infections, discharge and its characteristics, tinnitus, or vertigo.
   Health Promotion: Hearing loss, hearing aid use, how loss affects daily life, any exposure to environmental noise, method of cleaning ears.

Nose and Sinuses: Discharge and its characteristics, any unusually frequent or severe colds, sinus pain, nasal obstruction, nosebleeds, allergies or hay fever, or change in sense of smell.

Mouth and Throat: Mouth pain, frequent sore throat, bleeding gums, toothache, lesion in mouth or tongue, dysphagia, hoarseness or voice change, tonsillectomy, altered taste.
   Health Promotion: Pattern of daily dental care, use of prostheses (dentures, bridge), and last dental checkup.

Neck: Pain, limitation of motion, lumps or swelling, enlarged or tender nodes, goiter.

Breast: Pain, lump, nipple discharge, rash, history of breast disease, any surgery on breasts.
   Axilla: Tenderness, lump or swelling, rash.
   Health Promotion: Performs breast self-examination, including its frequency and method used, last mammogram and results.

(Circle if present.)   (Describe circled items.)

Respiratory System: History of lung disease (asthma, emphysema, bronchitis, pneumonia, tuberculosis), chest pain with breathing, wheezing or noisy breathing, shortness of breath, how much activity produces shortness of breath, cough, sputum (color, amount), hemoptysis, toxin or pollution exposure.
   Health Promotion: Last chest x-ray examination.

Cardiovascular System: Precordial or retrosternal pain, palpitation, cyanosis, dyspnea on exertion (specify amount of exertion it takes to produce dyspnea), orthopnea, paroxysmal nocturnal dyspnea, nocturia, edema, history of heart murmur, hypertension, coronary artery disease, anemia.
   Health Promotion: Date of last ECG or other heart tests and results.

Peripheral Vascular System: Coldness, numbness and tingling, swelling of legs (time of day, activity), discoloration in hands or feet (bluish red, pallor, mottling, associated with position, especially around feet and ankles), varicose veins or complications, intermittent claudication, thrombophlebitis, ulcers.
   Health Promotion: If work involves long-term sitting or standing, avoid crossing legs at the knees, wear support hose.

Gastrointestinal System: Appetite, food intolerance, dysphagia, heartburn, indigestion, pain (associated with eating), other abdominal pain, pyrosis (esophageal and stomach burning sensation with sour eructation), nausea and vomiting (character), vomiting blood, history of abdominal disease (ulcer, liver or gallbladder, jaundice, appendicitis, colitis), flatulence, frequency of bowel movement, any recent change, stool characteristics, constipation or diarrhea, black stools, rectal bleeding, rectal conditions, hemorrhoids, fistula).
   Health Promotion: Use of antacids or laxatives.

Urinary System: Frequency, urgency, nocturia (the number of times the person awakens at night to urinate, recent change), dysuria, polyuria or oliguria, hesitancy or straining, narrowed stream, urine color (cloudy or presence of hematuria), incontinence, history of urinary disease (kidney disease, kidney stones, urinary tract infections, prostate); pain in flank, groin, suprapubic region, or low back.
   Health Promotion: Measures to avoid or treat urinary tract infections, use of Kegel exercises after childbirth.

Male Genital System: Penis or testicular pain, sores or lesions, penile discharge, lumps, hernia.
   Health Promotion: Perform testicular self-examination? How frequently?

Female Genital System: Menstrual history (age at menarche, last menstrual period, cycle and duration, any amenorrhea or menorrhagia, premenstrual pain or dysmenorrhea, intermenstrual spotting), vaginal itching, discharge and its characteristics, age at menopause, menopausal signs or symptoms, post-menopausal bleeding.
   Health Promotion: Last gynecologic checkup, last Pap smear and results.

(Circle if present.)   (Describe circled items.)

Sexual Health: Presently in a relationship involving intercourse? Are aspects of sex satisfactory to you and partner, any dyspareunia (for female), any changes in erection or ejaculation (for male), use of contraceptive, is contraceptive method satisfactory? Use of condoms, how frequently? Aware of any contact with partner who has sexually transmitted infection (gonorrhea, herpes, chlamydia, venereal warts, HIV/AIDS, syphilis)?

Musculoskeletal System: History of arthritis or gout. In the joints: pain, stiffness, swelling (location, migratory nature), deformity, limitation of motion, noise with joint motion. In the muscles: any pain, cramps, weakness, gait problems or problems with coordinated activities. In the back: any pain (location and radiation to extremities), stiffness, limitation of motion, or history of back pain or disk disease.

> **Health Promotion:** How much walking per day. What is the effect of limited range of motion on daily activities, such as on grooming, feeding, toileting, dressing? Any mobility aids used?

Neurologic System: History of seizure disorder, stroke, fainting, blackouts. In motor function: weakness, tic or tremor, paralysis, coordination problems. In sensory function: numbness and tingling (paresthesia). In cognitive function: memory disorder (recent or distant, disorientation). In mental status: any nervousness, mood change, depression, or any history of mental health dysfunction or hallucinations.

Hematologic System: Bleeding tendency of skin or mucous membranes, excessive bruising, lymph node swelling, exposure to toxic agents or radiation, blood transfusion and reactions.

Endocrine System: History of diabetes or diabetic symptoms (polyuria, polydipsia, polyphagia), history of thyroid disease, intolerance to heat or cold, change in skin pigmentation or texture, excessive sweating, relationship between appetite and weight, abnormal hair distribution, nervousness, tremors, need for hormone therapy.

Functional Assessment (Including Activities of Daily Living)

Self-Esteem, Self-Concept: Education (last grade completed, other significant training) _____

_____

Financial status (income adequate for lifestyle and/or health concerns) _____

_____

Value-belief system (religious practices and perception of personal strengths) _____

_____

Self-care behaviors _____

_____

Activity/Exercise: Daily profile, usual pattern of a typical day _____

_____

Independent or needs assistance with ADLs, feeding, bathing, hygiene, dressing, toileting, bed-to-chair transfer, walking, standing, climbing stairs _____

_____

Leisure activities _____

Exercise pattern (type, amount per day or week, method of warm-up session, method of monitoring body's response to exercise) _____

_____

Other self-care behaviors _____

Sleep/Rest: Sleep patterns, daytime naps, any sleep aids used _____

_____

Other self-care behavior _____

Nutrition/Elimination: Record 24-hour diet recall _____

_____

Is this menu pattern typical of most days? _____

Who buys food? _____ Who prepares food? _____

Finances adequate for food? _____

Who is present at mealtimes? _____

Other self-care behaviors _____

Interpersonal Relationships/Resources: Describe own role in family _____

How getting along with family, friends, co-workers, classmates _____

_____

Get support with a problem from _____

How much daily time spent alone? _____

Is this pleasurable or isolating? _____

Other self-care behaviors _____

Coping and Stress Management: Describe stresses in life now _____

_____

Change in past year _____

Methods used to relieve stress _____

Are these methods helpful? _____

Personal Habits: Daily intake caffeine (coffee, tea, colas) _____

Smoke cigarettes? _____ Number packs per day _____

Daily use for how many years _____ Age started _____

Ever tried to quit? _____ How did it go? _____

Drink alcohol? _____ Date last alcohol use _____

Amount of alcohol that episode _____

Out of last 30 days, on how many days had alcohol? _____

Ever had a drinking problem? _____

Any use of street drugs? _____

Marijuana? _____ Cocaine? _____

Crack cocaine? _____ Amphetamines? _____

Barbiturates? _____ LSD? _____

Heroin? _____ Other? _____

Ever been in treatment for drugs or alcohol? _____

Environment/Hazards: Housing and neighborhood (type of structure, live alone, know neighbors) _____

_____

Safety of area _____

Adequate heat and utilities _____

Access to transportation _____

Involvement in community services _____

Hazards at workplace or home _____

Use of seatbelts _____

Travel to or residence in other countries _____

Military service in other countries _____

Self-care behaviors _____

Intimate Partner Violence: How are things at home? Do you feel safe? _____

_____

Ever been emotionally or physically abused by your partner or someone important to you? _____

Ever been hit, slapped, kicked, pushed, or shoved or otherwise physically hurt by your partner or ex-partner?

_____

Partner ever force you into having sex? _____

Are you afraid of your partner or ex-partner? _____

Occupational Health: Please describe your job _____

Work with any health hazards (e.g., asbestos, inhalants, chemicals, repetitive motion)? _____

_____

Any equipment at work designed to reduce your exposure? _____

Any work programs designed to monitor your exposure? _____

Any health problems that you think are related to your job? _____

What do you like or dislike about your job? _____

Perception of Own Health: How do you define health? _____

View of own health now _____

What are your concerns? _____

What do you expect will happen to your health in future? _____

_____

Your health goals _____

Your expectations of nurses, physicians _____

Mental Status Assessment

PURPOSE

This chapter helps you learn the components of the mental status examination, including assessing a person's appearance, behavior, cognitive functions, and thought processes and perceptions; understand the rationale and methods of examination of mental status; and record the assessment accurately.

READING ASSIGNMENT

Jarvis: *Physical Examination and Health Assessment*, 6th ed., Chapter 5, pp. 71-92.

GLOSSARY

Study the following terms after completing the reading assignment. You should be able to cover the definition on the right and define the term out loud.

Abstract reasoning . . . . pondering a deeper meaning beyond the concrete and literal

Attention . . . . concentration, ability to focus on one specific thing

Consciousness . . . . being aware of one's own existence, feelings, and thoughts and being aware of the environment

Delirium . . . . an acute confusional change or loss of consciousness and perceptual disturbance, may accompany acute illness, and usually resolves when the underlying cause is treated

Dementia . . . . a gradual progressive process, causing decreased cognitive function even though the person is fully conscious and awake, and is not reversible

Language . . . . using the voice to communicate one's thoughts and feelings

Memory . . . . ability to lay down and store experiences and perceptions for later recall

Mood . . . . prolonged display of a person's feelings

Orientation . . . . awareness of the objective world in relation to the self

Perceptions . . . . awareness of objects through any of the five senses

Thought content . . . . *what* the person thinks—specific ideas, beliefs, the use of words

Thought process . . . . the *way* a person thinks, the logical train of thought

STUDY GUIDE

After completing the reading assignment, you should be able to answer the following questions in the spaces provided.

1. Define the term *mental disorder*.

2. Differentiate *organic brain disorder* from *psychiatric mental illness*.

3. List 4 situations in which it would be necessary to perform a complete mental status examination.

4. Explain 4 factors that could affect a patient's response to the mental status examination but have nothing to do with mental disorders.

5. Distinguish *dysphonia* from *dysarthria*.

6. Define *unilateral neglect*, and state the illness with which it is associated.

7. State convenient ways to assess a person's recent memory within the context of the initial health history.

8. Which mental function is the Four Unrelated Words Test intended to test?

9. List at least 3 questions you could ask a patient that would screen for suicide ideation.

10. Describe the patient response level of consciousness that would be graded as:

Lethargic or somnolent _____

Obtunded _____

Stupor or semi-coma _____

Coma _____

Delirium _____

REVIEW QUESTIONS

This test is for you to check your own mastery of the content. Answers are provided in Appendix A.

1. Although a full mental status examination may not be required, you must be aware of the four main headings of the assessment while performing the interview and physical examination. These headings are:

   a. mood, affect, consciousness, and orientation.
   b. memory, attention, thought content, and perceptions.
   c. language, orientation, attention, and abstract reasoning.
   d. appearance, behavior, cognition, and thought processes.

2. Select the finding that most accurately describes the appearance of a patient.

   a. Tense posture and restless activity. Clothing clean but not appropriate for season (e.g., patient wearing T-shirt and shorts in cold weather).
   b. Oriented × 3. Affect appropriate for circumstances.
   c. Alert and responds to verbal stimuli. Tearful when diagnosis discussed.
   d. Laughing inappropriately, oriented × 3.

3. The ability to lay down new memories is part of the assessment of cognitive functions. One way to accomplish this is by:

   a. noting whether the patient completes a thought without wandering.
   b. a test of general knowledge.
   c. a description of past medical history.
   d. use of the Four Unrelated Words Test.

4. To accurately plan for discharge teaching, additional assessments may be required for the patient with aphasia. This may be accomplished by asking the patient to:

   a. calculate serial 7s.
   b. name his or her grandchildren and their birthdays.
   c. demonstrate word comprehension by naming articles in the room or on the body as you point to them.
   d. interpret a proverb.

5. During an interview with a patient newly diagnosed with a seizure disorder, the patient states, "I plan to be an airline pilot." If the patient continues to have this as a career goal after teaching regarding seizure disorders has been provided, the practitioner might question the patient's:

   a. thought processes.
   b. judgment.
   c. attention span.
   d. recent memory.

6. On a patient's second day in an acute care hospital, the patient complains about the "bugs" on the bed. The bed is clean. This would be an example of altered:

   a. thought process.
   b. orientation.
   c. perception.
   d. higher intellectual function.

7. One way to assess cognitive function and to detect dementia is with:

   a. the Proverb Interpretation Test.
   b. the Mini-Cog.
   c. the Denver II.
   d. the Older Adult Behavioral Checklist.

8. The Behavioral Checklist by Jellinek, Evans, and Knight (1979; see Table 5-2 in Jarvis: *Physical Examination and Health Assessment*, 4th ed., p. 79), which is completed by a parent, is used to assess the mental status of:

   a. infants.
   b. children 1 to 5 years of age.
   c. children 7 to 11 years of age.
   d. adolescents.

9. A major characteristic of dementia is:

   a. impairment of short- and long-term memory.
   b. hallucinations.
   c. sudden onset of symptoms.
   d. substance-induced.

10. Which of the following is an example of a patient with dysarthria?

    a. When asked a question, the patient responds fluently but uses words incorrectly or makes up words so that speech may be incomprehensible.
    b. The word choice and grammar are appropriate, but the sounds are distorted so speech is unintelligible.
    c. The pitch and volume of words are difficult and the voice may be hoarse, but language is intact.
    d. Comprehension is intact but there is difficulty in expressing thoughts, with nouns and verbs being the dominant word choices.

11. The nurse is leading a discussion of the planned activities for the day at an adult living center and states, "We will be having snacks at 9:30 and lunch will be at noon." One of the participants responds in a very monotone manner, "Snacks at 9:30, lunch at noon, snacks at 9:30, lunch at noon." This patient is exhibiting signs of:

    a. echolalia.
    b. confabulation.
    c. flight of ideas.
    d. neologisms.

Match column B to column A.

Column A—Definition

12. ___ Lack of emotional response

13. ___ Loss of identity

14. ___ Excessive well-being

15. ___ Apprehensive from the anticipation of a danger whose source is unknown

16. ___ Annoyed, easily provoked

17. ___ Loss of control

18. ___ Sad, gloomy, dejected

19. ___ Rapid shift of emotions

20. ___ Worried about known external danger

Column B—Type of mood and affect

a. Depression

b. Anxiety

c. Flat affect

d. Euphoria

e. Lability

f. Rage

g. Irritability

h. Fear

i. Depersonalization

21. Write a narrative account of a mental status assessment with normal findings.

SKILLS LABORATORY/CLINICAL SETTING

You are now ready for the clinical component of the mental status examination. The purpose of the clinical component is to achieve beginning competency with the administration of the mental status examination and with the supplemental Mini-Mental State Examination.

Practice the steps of the full mental status examination on a peer or a patient in the clinical setting, giving appropriate instructions as you proceed. Formulate ahead of time your questions to pose to the patient. Record your findings using the regional write-up sheet that follows.

Next, practice the steps of the Mini-Mental State Examination, which is a simplified scored form of the cognitive functions found on the full mental status examination. It is used frequently in clinical and research settings.

NOTES

REGIONAL WRITE-UP—MENTAL STATUS EXAMINATION

Date _____

Examiner _____

Patient _____ Age _____ Gender _____

Occupation _____

Mental Status
(Before testing, tell the person the four words you want him or her to remember and to recall in a few minutes, for the Four Unrelated Words Test.)

1. **Appearance**

   Posture _____
   Body movements _____
   Dress _____
   Grooming and hygiene _____

2. **Behavior**

   Level of consciousness _____
   Facial expression _____
   Speech:
      Quality _____
      Pace _____
      Word choice _____
   Mood and affect _____

3. **Cognitive Functions**

   Orientation:
      Time _____
      Place _____
      Person _____
   Attention span _____
   Recent memory _____
   Remote memory _____
   New learning—Four Unrelated Words Test _____
   Additional testing for aphasia:
      Word comprehension _____
      Reading _____
      Writing _____
   Judgment _____

4. **Thought Processes and Perceptions**

   Thought processes _____
   Thought content _____
   Perceptions _____
   Suicidal thoughts _____

Mini-Mental State Examination (MMSE)

Sample Items

Orientation to Time

"What is the date?"

Registration

"Listen carefully, I am going to say three words. You say them back after I stop. Ready? Here they are..."

HOUSE (pause), CAR (pause), LAKE (pause). Now repeat those words back to me." [Repeat up to 5 times, but score only the first trial.]

Naming

"What is this?" [Point to a pencil or pen.]

Reading

"Please read this and do what it says." [Show examinee the words on the stimulus form.]

For a full copy of the MMSE, administration instructions, and scoring guidelines, contact Psychological Assessment Resources, ©1975, 1998, 2001 by MiniMental, LLC. All rights reserved. Published 2001 by Psychological Assessment Resources, Inc. May not be reproduced in whole or in part in any form or by any means without written permission of the Psychological Assessment Resources, Inc., 16204 N. Florida Ave., Lutz, FL 33549; telephone 1-800-331-8378 or 813-968-3003; website: *www.Minimental.com.* From Folstein et al, 1985.

Substance Use Assessment

PURPOSE

This chapter presents the scope of the problem regarding primary care and hospital patients who drink excessive alcohol and use illicit drugs. Screening tools and interview approaches are presented.

READING ASSIGNMENT

Jarvis: *Physical Examination and Health Assessment*, 6th ed., Chapter 6, pp. 93-102.

GLOSSARY

Study the following terms after completing the reading assignment. You should be able to cover the definition on the right and define the term out loud.

Alcohol abuse . . . . one or more of the following events in a year: recurrent use resulting in failure to fulfill major role obligations; recurrent use in hazardous situations; recurrent alcohol-related legal problems (e.g., DUI); continued use despite social or interpersonal problems caused or exacerbated by alcohol

Alcohol dependence . . . . three or more of the following events in a year: tolerance (increased amounts to achieve effect; diminished effect from same amount); withdrawal; a great deal of time spent obtaining alcohol, using it, or recovering from its effect; important activities given up or reduced because of alcohol; drinking more or longer than intended; persistent desire or unsuccessful efforts to cut down or control alcohol use; use continued despite knowledge of having a psychological problem caused or exacerbated by alcohol

At-risk drinking . . . . Men, 14 or more drinks/week or 4 or more drinks/occasion; Women, 7 or more drinks/week or 3 or more drinks/occasion

STUDY GUIDE

After completing the reading assignment, you should be able to answer the following questions in the space provided.

1. What proportion of Americans ages 12 and older report being current alcohol drinkers? And report being binge drinkers (≥5 drinks/occasion)?

2. List the effects of alcohol on 4 traumatic or disease conditions.

3. Define the use of prescription opioid pain relievers for a nonmedical use.

4. Discuss the extra risk alcohol drinking poses to the aging adult.

5. Contrast the use and settings for the following alcohol screening tools: AUDIT; AUDIT-C; CAGE questionnaire.

6. State 3 clinical laboratory findings that are used to detect or monitor alcohol use.

ADDITIONAL LEARNING ACTIVITIES

1. Read your daily newspaper for 1 week, making a list of all news stories (auto accidents, drowning, personal injury, etc.) that are or possibly could be alcohol-related.

2. In a group of 3 or 4 students, interview a primary care physician, emergency department physician, and intensive care unit physician. Ask each one for clinical examples of alcohol-related cases in their units.

3. Attend one open meeting of Alcoholics Anonymous. Enter your zip code in the AA website (*www.aa.org*) to find locations. Be fully aware of the anonymous tradition of these meetings, and do not repeat any personal information.

4. Look up your school's/university's alcohol policy in your student handbook. Possibly the ideal handbook statement is different from the actual situation on your campus. How is this different?

REVIEW QUESTIONS

This test is for you to check your own mastery of the content. Answers are provided in Appendix A.

1. As defined by the American Psychiatric Association DSM-IV criteria, which of the following is characterized by, for example, a college student's (1) failure to attend class and complete assignments, (2) driving while intoxicated, (3) legal problems such as a DUI, and (4) continued use despite problems?

   a. Drug dependence
   b. Drug habituation
   c. Relief drug use
   d. Drug abuse

2. The phase of addiction characterized by tolerance, increasing time spent in substance-related activities, unsuccessful attempts to quit, and continued use despite known harm is:

   a. relief.
   b. withdrawal.
   c. dependency.
   d. preoccupation.

3. The unpleasant effect that occurs when use of a drug is stopped is called:

   a. potency.
   b. withdrawal.
   c. metabolism.
   d. threshold.

4. The need for increasingly larger doses of a substance to achieve the same effect that was initially experienced from using is called:

   a. tolerance.
   b. addiction.
   c. abuse.
   d. dependence.

5. Prolonged heavy drinking can lead to all of the following *except:*

   a. kidney and liver damage.
   b. increased risk of oral cancer.
   c. increased resistance to pneumonia and other infectious diseases.
   d. damage to brain and peripheral nervous system.

6. How many drinks does a person consume in one sitting for it to be considered binge drinking?

   a. 3
   b. 5
   c. 7
   d. 8

7. A pregnant woman explains to the examiner that she does not intend to stop drinking because several of her friends continued to drink during pregnancy and "nothing happened to them or their kids." How should the examiner respond to this statement?

   a. "While it's true that there is no scientific evidence that alcohol harms the fetus, abstinence is recommended because of the physical effects on your body."
   b. "No amount of alcohol has been determined to be safe for a pregnant women so I would like to ask you to stop drinking alcohol completely."
   c. "Maybe you could cut back on your alcohol intake, at least until you're in the third trimester when the effects on the fetus are minimal."
   d. "If you can limit yourself to only one drink per day, you will be helping yourself and your baby."

8. Which is the most commonly used laboratory test to identify chronic alcohol drinking?

   a. blood urea nitrogen
   b. liver enzyme panel
   c. gamma glutamyl transferase (GGT)
   d. mean corpuscular volume (MCV)

NOTES

Domestic Violence Assessment

PURPOSE

This chapter helps you learn about intimate partner violence, elder abuse, and child abuse. The content includes how to assess the extent of the abuse, how to assess the extent of physical and psychological harm, and how to document appropriately.

READING ASSIGNMENT

Jarvis: *Physical Examination and Health Assessment*, 6th ed., Chapter 7, pp. 103-114.

GLOSSARY

Study the following terms after completing the reading assignment. You should be able to cover the definition on the right and define the term out loud.

Child emotional abuse . . . . any pattern of behavior that harms a child's emotional development or sense of self-worth. It includes frequent belittling, rejection, threats, and withholding love and support

Child neglect . . . . failure to provide for a child's basic needs (physical, educational, medical, and emotional)

Child physical abuse . . . . physical injury due to punching, beating, kicking, biting, burning, shaking, or otherwise harming a child. Even if the parent or caregiver did not intend to harm the child, such acts are considered abuse when done purposefully

Child sexual abuse . . . . includes fondling a child's genitals, incest, penetration, rape, sodomy, indecent exposure, and commercial exploitation through prostitution or the production of pornographic materials

Elder abuse . . . . willful infliction of force that results in bodily harm, pain, and/or impairment on a person age 65 years or older. Examples include pushing, slapping, hitting, shaking, burning, and rough handling

Elder neglect (physical) . . . . . . physical harm (actual or potential) to person age 65 years or older because of failure to provide for the person's well-being. Examples include inadequate feeding and hydration, unsanitary living conditions, and poor personal hygiene

**Intimate partner
violence (IPV)** . . . . physical and/or sexual violence (use of physical force) or threat of such violence; also psychological/emotional abuse and/or coercive tactics when there has been prior physical and/or sexual violence between spouses or non-marital partners (dating, boyfriend-girlfriend) or former spouses or non-marital partners

**Mandatory reporting
of abuse** . . . . a specified group of people (e.g., health care providers) is required by law to report abuse (of a specified nature against specified people) to a governmental agency (e.g., protective services, the police)

Psychological abuse . . . . infliction of emotional/mental anguish by humiliation, coercion, and threats and/or lack of social stimulation. Examples include yelling, threats of harm, threats of withholding basic medical and/or personal care, and leaving the person alone for long periods

**Routine universal
screening for intimate
partner violence** . . . . asking all adult patients (usually female patients) each time they are in the health care system, no matter what their problem or concern, whether they have experienced IPV

STUDY GUIDE

After completing the reading assignment, you should be able to answer the following questions in the spaces provided.

1. Identify the most common physical health problems that result from intimate partner violence.

2. Identify the most common mental health problems that result from intimate partner violence.

3. Differentiate abuse from neglect.

4. Identify commonly used screening questions for intimate partner violence.

5. Identify commonly used screening questions for older adult abuse.

6. Differentiate routine universal screening from indicator-based screening.

7. Identify important elements of assessment for an abused person.

8. List 2 potential sources of lethality in intimate partner violence situations.

9. Discuss bruising in children and how it relates to their development level.

10. Identify some of the important elements of the child's medical history when assessing for suspected child maltreatment.

11. Discuss some of the long-term consequences of child maltreatment.

12. Identify risk factors that may contribute to child maltreatment.

ADDITIONAL LEARNING ACTIVITIES

1. Read your daily newspaper for a month, cutting out stories that are related to intimate partner (domestic) violence, elder abuse, including stories about intimate partner or elder homicide, or child maltreatment. Notice details of the story, including if there is subtle "victim blaming," various myths about abuse that are apparent, or precipitating factors that are identified.

2. Recall whether you were asked about intimate partner violence at your last encounter as a patient in the health care system. Check to see if your health care provider has any posters about domestic violence or brochures in the restrooms or other accessible areas.

3. Visit your local shelter for domestic violence. Take note of what health care services are offered to women and children who are staying there. Take note of volunteer opportunities, and tell your friends about them.

4. Visit your local adult protective services/child protective services office. Find out what happens when a nurse makes a report about elder/child abuse.

5. Find out what your state laws are about mandatory reporting of intimate partner violence and elder abuse. See if your clinical practice site has policies and procedures that match the state law.

REVIEW QUESTIONS

This test is for you to check your own mastery of the content. Answers are provided in Appendix A.

1. Which of the following are examples of intimate partner violence?

   a. an ex-boyfriend stalks his ex-girlfriend
   b. marital rape
   c. hitting a date
   d. all of the above

2. Routine universal screening for domestic violence means:

   a. asking all women each time they come to the health care system if they are abused.
   b. asking women who have injuries if they are abused.
   c. asking women who have symptoms of depression and PTSD if they are abused.
   d. asking women ages 18 to 30 years if they are abused.

3. Mental health problems associated with intimate partner violence include:

   a. hallucinations.
   b. suicidality.
   c. schizophrenia.
   d. attention deficit/hyperactivity disorder (ADHD).

4. Gynecologic problems *not* associated with intimate partner violence include:

   a. pelvic pain.
   b. ovarian cysts.
   c. STIs.
   d. vaginal tearing.

5. Risk factors for intimate partner homicide include:

   a. abuse during pregnancy.
   b. victim substance abuse.
   c. victim unemployment.
   d. history of victim childhood sexual assault.

6. Elder abuse and neglect include:

   a. willful infliction of force.
   b. withholding prescription medications without medical orders.
   c. not replacing broken eyeglasses.
   d. threatening to place someone in a nursing home.
   e. all of the above.

7. When assessing an injury on a child, which of the following should be considered?

   a. the child's developmental level
   b. the child's medical and medication history
   c. the history of how the injury occurred
   d. all of the above

8. Known risk factors for child maltreatment include which of the following?

   a. substance abuse
   b. intimate partner violence
   c. physical disability/mental retardation in the child
   d. all of the above

9. Bruising in a non-walking or non-cruising child:

   a. is a common finding from normal infant activity.
   b. needs to be further evaluated for either an abusive or medical explanation.
   c. is commonly seen on the buttocks.
   d. cannot be reported until after a full medical evaluation.

10. Which of the following is a forensic term that is related to "purpura" but is not related to blunt force trauma?

    a. wound
    b. incision
    c. ecchymosis
    d. bruise

11. Which of the following should be routinely included in evaluating a case of elder abuse?

    a. corroborative interview from caregiver
    b. baseline laboratory tests
    c. testing for STIs
    d. TB test

NOTES

CHAPTER
8

Assessment Techniques and the Clinical Setting

PURPOSE

This chapter helps you learn the assessment techniques of inspection, palpation, percussion, and auscultation; learn the items of equipment needed for a complete physical examination; and consider age-specific modifications you would make for the examination of individuals throughout the life cycle.

READING ASSIGNMENT

Jarvis: *Physical Examination and Health Assessment*, 6th ed., Chapter 8, pp. 115-126.

GLOSSARY

Study the following terms after completing the reading assignment. You should be able to cover the definition on the right and define the term out loud.

Amplitude . . . . (or intensity) how loud or soft a sound is

Duration . . . . the length of time a note lingers

Nosocomial infection . . . . an infection acquired during hospitalization

Ophthalmoscope . . . . an instrument that illuminates the internal eye structures, enabling the examiner to look through the pupil at the fundus (background) of the eye

Otoscope . . . . an instrument that illuminates the ear canal, enabling the examiner to look at the ear canal and tympanic membrane

Pitch . . . . (or frequency) the number of vibrations (or cycles) per second of a note

Quality . . . . (or timbre) a subjective difference in a sound due to the sound's distinctive overtones

STUDY GUIDE

After completing the reading assignment, you should be able to answer the following questions in the spaces provided.

1. Define and describe the technique of the 4 physical examination skills:

   Inspection _____

   Palpation _____

   Percussion _____

   Auscultation _____

2. Define the characteristics of the following percussion notes:

	Pitch	Amplitude	Quality	Duration
Resonance				
Hyperresonance				
Tympany				
Dull				
Flat				

3. Relate the parts of the hands to palpation techniques used in assessment.

4. Differentiate between light, deep, and bimanual palpation.

5. List the two endpieces of the stethoscope and the conditions for which each is best suited.

6. Describe the environmental conditions to consider in preparing the examination setting.

7. List the 20 basic items of equipment necessary to conduct a complete physical examination on an adult.

8. List 4 situations in which you clean your hands promptly and thoroughly.

9. Describe your own preparation as you encounter the patient for examination: your own dress, your demeanor, safety/Universal Precautions, sequence of examination steps, instructions to patient.

10. What age-specific considerations would you make for the examination of the:

Infant? _____

Toddler? _____

Preschooler? _____

School-age child? _____

Adolescent? _____

Older adult? _____

Acutely ill person? _____

_____

Note that six tables summarizing growth and development milestones for infancy through adolescence can be found in the appendixes of this Student Laboratory Manual, for your reference.

REVIEW QUESTIONS

This test is for you to check your own mastery of the content. Answers are provided in Appendix A.

1. Various parts of the hands are used during palpation. The part of the hand used for the assessment of vibration is (are) the:

   a. fingertips.
   b. index finger and thumb in opposition.
   c. dorsum of the hand.
   d. ulnar surface of the hand.

2. When performing indirect percussion, the stationary finger is struck:

   a. at the ulnar surface.
   b. at the middle joint.
   c. at the distal interphalangeal joint.
   d. wherever it is in contact with the skin.

3. The best description of the pitch of a sound wave obtained by percussion is:

   a. the intensity of the sound.
   b. the number of vibrations per second.
   c. the length of time the note lingers.
   d. the overtones of the note.

4. The bell of the stethoscope:

   a. is used for soft, low-pitched sounds.
   b. is used for high-pitched sounds.
   c. is held firmly against the skin.
   d. magnifies sound.

5. The ophthalmoscope has 5 apertures. Which aperture would be used to assess the eyes of a patient with undilated pupils?

   a. grid
   b. slit
   c. small
   d. large

6. At the conclusion of the examination, the examiner should:

   a. document findings before leaving the examining room.
   b. have findings confirmed by another practitioner.
   c. relate objective findings to the subjective findings for accuracy.
   d. summarize findings to the patient.

7. When the practitioner enters the examining room, the infant patient is asleep. The practitioner would best start the examination with:

   a. height and weight.
   b. blood pressure.
   c. heart, lung, and abdomen.
   d. temperature.

8. The sequence of an examination changes from beginning with the thorax to that of head to toe with what age child?

   a. the infant
   b. the preschool child
   c. the school-age child
   d. the adolescent

9. When inspecting the ear canal, the examiner chooses which speculum for the otoscope?

   a. a short, broad one
   b. the narrowest for a child
   c. the longest for an adult
   d. the largest that will fit

10. A nosocomial infection is one that is acquired:

    a. in a hospital setting.
    b. in a public facility.
    c. by the fecal-oral route.
    d. through airborne contaminants.

SKILLS LABORATORY/CLINICAL SETTING

Note that the clinical component of this chapter is combined with Chapter 9. Instructions and regional write-up forms are listed at the end of Chapter 9.

General Survey, Measurement, Vital Signs

PURPOSE

This chapter helps you learn the method of gathering data for a general survey on a patient and the techniques for measuring height, weight, body mass index, and vital signs.

READING ASSIGNMENT

Jarvis: *Physical Examination and Health Assessment,* 6th ed., Chapter 9, pp. 127-158.

GLOSSARY

Study the following terms after completing the reading assignment. You should be able to cover the definition on the right and define the term out loud.

Auscultatory gap . . . . a brief time period when Korotkoff sounds disappear during auscultation of blood pressure; common with hypertension

Bradycardia. . . . . heart rate <50 beats per minute in the adult

Sphygmomanometer. . . . . instrument for measuring arterial blood pressure

Stroke volume . . . . amount of blood pumped out of the heart with each heartbeat

Tachycardia. . . . . heart rate of >90 beats per minute in the adult

STUDY GUIDE

After completing the reading assignment, you should be able to answer the following questions in the spaces provided.

1. List the significant information considered in each of the 4 areas of a general survey—physical appearance, body structure, mobility, and behavior.

2. Describe the normal posture and body build.

3. Note aspects of normal gait.

4. Describe the clinical appearance of the following variations in stature:

   Hypopituitary dwarfism _____

   Gigantism _____

   Acromegaly _____

   Achondroplastic dwarfism _____

   Marfan syndrome _____

   Endogenous obesity (Cushing syndrome) _____

   Anorexia nervosa _____

5. State the body mass index for a male weighing 190 lbs and 5'10" tall _____; for a female weighing 136 lbs and 5'4" tall _____.

6. For serial weight measurements, what time of day would you instruct the person to have the weight measured?

7. Describe the technique for measuring head circumference and chest circumference on an infant.

8. What changes in height and in weight distribution would you expect for an adult in his or her 70s and 80s?

9. Describe the tympanic membrane thermometer, and compare its use with other forms of temperature measurement.

10. Describe 3 qualities to consider when assessing the pulse.

11. Relate the qualities of normal respirations to the appropriate approach to counting them.

12. Define and describe the relationships among the terms *blood pressure, systolic pressure, diastolic pressure, pulse pressure,* and *mean arterial pressure.*

13. List factors that affect blood pressure.

14. Relate the use of the wrong size blood pressure cuff to the possible findings that may be obtained.

15. Explain the significance of phase I, phase IV, and phase V Korotkoff sounds during blood pressure measurement.

16. Given an apparently healthy 20-year-old adult, state the expected range for oral temperature, pulse, respirations, and blood pressure.

17. List the parameters of prehypertension, stage 1 hypertension, and stage 2 hypertension.

REVIEW QUESTIONS

This test is for you to check your own mastery of the content. Answers are provided in Appendix A.

1. The 4 areas to consider during the general survey are:
   a. ethnicity, gender, age, and socioeconomic status.
   b. physical appearance, gender, ethnicity, and affect.
   c. dress, affect, nonverbal behavior, and mobility.
   d. physical appearance, body structure, mobility, and behavior.

2. During the general survey part of the examination, gait is assessed. When walking, the base is usually:
   a. varied, depending on the height of the person.
   b. equal to the length of the arm.
   c. as wide as the shoulder width.
   d. half the height of the person.

3. An 18-month-old child is brought in for a health screening visit. To assess the height of the child:

   a. use a tape measure.
   b. use a horizontal measuring board.
   c. have the child stand on the upright scale.
   d. measure arm span to estimate height.

4. What changes in head circumference measurements in relation to chest measurements will occur from infancy through early childhood?

   a. A newborn's head should be about 5 cm larger than the chest circumference, but by age 2, they should be equal.
   b. The chest grows at a faster rate than the cranium, but at age 1, the measurements will be the same, and after age 2, the chest should be about 5 cm larger.
   c. The newborn's head will be 2 cm larger than the chest circumference, but between 6 months and 2 years, they will be about the same.
   d. The head and chest circumferences should be very similar, but between 6 months and 2 years, the chest size will increase and remain that way.

5. During the 8th and 9th decades of life, physical changes occur. Height and weight:

   a. both increase.
   b. weight increases, height decreases.
   c. both decrease.
   d. both remain the same as during the 70s.

6. During an initial home visit, the patient's temperature is noted to be 97.4° F. This temperature:

   a. cannot be evaluated without a knowledge of the person's age.
   b. is below normal. The person should be assessed for possible hypothermia.
   c. should be retaken by the rectal route, since this best reflects core body temperature.
   d. should be reevaluated at the next visit before a decision is made.

7. Select the best description of an accurate assessment of a patient's pulse.

   a. Count for 15 seconds if pulse is regular.
   b. Begin counting with zero; count for 30 seconds.
   c. Count for 30 seconds and multiply by 2 for all cases.
   d. Count for 1 full minute; begin counting with zero.

8. After assessing the patient's pulse, the practitioner determines it to be "normal." This would be recorded as:

   a. 3+.
   b. 2+.
   c. 1+.
   d. 0.

9. Select the best description of an accurate assessment of a patient's respirations.

   a. Count for a full minute before taking the pulse.
   b. Count for 15 seconds and multiply by 4.
   c. Count after informing the patient where you are in the assessment process.
   d. Count for 30 seconds after pulse assessment.

10. Pulse pressure is:

    a. the difference between the systolic and diastolic pressure.
    b. a reflection of the viscosity of the blood.
    c. another way to express the systolic pressure.
    d. a measure of vasoconstriction.

11. The examiner is going to assess for coarctation of the aorta. In an individual with coarctation, the thigh pressure would be:

    a. higher than in the arm.
    b. equal to that in the arm.
    c. unrelated to the arm pressure. There is no constant relationship; findings are highly individual.
    d. lower than in the arm.

12. Mean arterial pressure is:

    a. the arithmetic average of systolic and diastolic pressures.
    b. the driving force of blood during systole.
    c. diastolic pressure plus one-third pulse pressure.
    d. corresponding to phase III Korotkoff.

13. Why is it important to match the appropriate-size blood pressure cuff to the person's arm and shape and not to the person's age?

    a. Using a cuff that is too narrow will give a false reading that is high.
    b. Using a cuff that is too wide will give a false reading that is low.
    c. Using a cuff that is too narrow will give a false reading that is low.
    d. Using a cuff that is too wide will give a false reading that is high.

SKILLS LABORATORY/CLINICAL SETTING

You are now ready for the clinical component of Chapters 8 and 9. The purpose of the clinical component is to observe and describe the regional examination on a peer in the skills laboratory and to achieve the following.

Clinical Objectives

1. Observe and describe the significant characteristics of a general survey.

2. Measure height and weight, and determine if findings are within normal range.

3. Gather vital signs data.

4. Record the physical examination findings accurately.

Instructions

Set up your section of the skills laboratory for a complete physical examination, attending to proper lighting, tables, and linen. Gather all equipment you will need for a complete physical examination, and make sure you are familiar with its mechanical operation. You will not use all the equipment today, but you will use it during the course of the semester and this is the time to have it checked out.

Practice the steps of gathering data for a general survey, for height and weight, and for vital signs on a peer. Record your findings using the regional write-up sheet that follows. The first section of the sheet is intended as a worksheet. It includes points for you to note that add up to the general survey. The bottom of the sheet has instructions for you to write the general survey statement; this is the topic sentence that will serve as an introduction for the complete physical examination write-up (see Jarvis: *Physical Examination and Health Assessment,* 6th ed., p. 153, for an example).

REGIONAL WRITE-UP—GENERAL SURVEY, VITAL SIGNS

Date _____

Examiner _____

Patient _____ Age _____ Gender _____

Occupation _____

I. Physical Examination
A. General survey
1. Physical appearance
   Age _____
   Gender _____
   Level of consciousness _____
   Skin color _____
   Facial features _____
2. Body structure
   Stature _____
   Nutrition _____
   Symmetry _____
   Posture _____
   Position _____
   Body build, contour _____
   Any physical deformity _____
3. Mobility
   Gait _____
   Range of motion _____
4. Behavior
   Facial expression _____
   Mood and affect _____
   Speech _____
   Dress _____
   Personal hygiene _____

B. Measurement
1. Height: _____ cm; _____ ft/inches   3. Body mass index _____
2. Weight: _____ kg; _____ lb   4. Waist circumference: inches _____

C. Vital signs
1. Temperature _____
2. Pulse _____
   Rate _____
   Rhythm _____
3. Respirations _____
4. Blood pressure: _____ R arm; _____ L arm

II. Summary
(Write a summary of the general survey, including height, weight, and vital signs. This will serve as an introduction for the complete physical examination write-up.)

TABLE 9-1 BODY MASS INDEX

BMI	Normal						Overweight					Obese									
	19	20	21	22	23	24	25	26	27	28	29	30	31	32	33	34	35	36	37	38	39
HEIGHT (INCHES)	**BODY WEIGHT (POUNDS)**																				
58	91	96	100	105	110	115	119	124	129	134	138	143	148	153	158	162	167	172	177	181	186
59	94	99	104	109	114	119	124	128	133	138	143	148	153	158	163	168	173	178	183	188	193
60	97	102	107	112	118	123	128	133	138	143	148	153	158	163	168	174	179	184	189	194	199
61	100	106	111	116	122	127	132	137	143	148	153	158	164	169	174	180	185	190	195	201	206
62	104	109	115	120	126	131	136	142	147	153	158	164	169	175	180	186	191	196	202	207	213
63	107	113	118	124	130	135	141	146	152	158	163	169	175	180	186	191	197	203	208	214	220
64	110	116	122	128	134	140	145	151	157	163	169	174	180	186	192	197	204	209	215	221	227
65	114	120	126	132	138	144	150	156	162	168	174	180	186	192	198	204	210	216	222	228	234
66	118	124	130	136	142	148	155	161	167	173	179	186	192	198	204	210	216	223	229	235	241
67	121	127	134	140	146	153	159	166	172	178	185	191	198	204	211	217	223	230	236	242	249
68	125	131	138	144	151	158	164	171	177	184	190	197	203	210	216	223	230	236	243	249	256
69	128	135	142	149	155	162	169	176	182	189	196	203	209	216	223	230	236	243	250	257	263
70	132	139	146	153	160	167	174	181	188	195	202	209	216	222	229	236	243	250	257	264	271
71	136	143	150	157	165	172	179	186	193	200	208	215	222	229	236	243	250	257	265	272	279
72	140	147	154	162	169	177	184	191	199	206	213	221	228	235	242	250	258	265	272	279	287
73	144	151	159	166	174	182	189	197	204	212	219	227	235	242	250	257	265	272	280	288	295
74	148	155	163	171	179	186	194	202	210	218	225	233	241	249	256	264	272	280	287	295	303
75	152	160	168	176	184	192	200	208	216	224	232	240	248	256	264	272	279	287	295	303	311
76	156	164	172	180	189	197	205	213	221	230	238	246	254	263	271	279	287	295	304	312	320

BMI	Extreme Obesity														
	40	41	42	43	44	45	46	47	48	49	50	51	52	53	54
HEIGHT (INCHES)	**BODY WEIGHT (POUNDS)**														
58	191	196	201	205	210	215	220	224	229	234	239	244	248	253	258
59	198	203	208	212	217	222	227	232	237	242	247	252	257	262	267
60	204	209	215	220	225	230	235	240	245	250	255	261	266	271	276
61	211	217	222	227	232	238	243	248	254	259	264	269	275	280	285
62	218	224	229	235	240	246	251	256	262	267	273	278	284	289	295
63	225	231	237	242	248	254	259	265	270	278	282	287	293	299	304
64	232	238	244	250	256	262	267	273	279	285	291	296	302	308	314
65	240	246	252	258	264	270	276	282	288	294	300	306	312	318	324
66	247	253	260	266	272	278	284	291	297	303	309	315	322	328	334
67	255	261	268	274	280	287	293	299	306	312	319	325	331	338	344
68	262	269	276	282	289	295	302	308	315	322	328	335	341	348	354
69	270	277	284	291	297	304	311	318	324	331	338	345	351	358	365
70	278	285	292	299	306	313	320	327	334	341	348	355	362	369	376
71	286	293	301	308	315	322	329	338	343	351	358	365	372	379	386
72	294	302	309	316	324	331	338	346	353	361	368	375	383	390	397
73	302	310	318	325	333	340	348	355	363	371	378	386	393	401	408
74	311	319	326	334	342	350	358	365	373	381	389	396	404	412	420
75	319	327	335	343	351	359	367	375	383	391	399	407	415	423	431
76	328	336	344	353	361	369	377	385	394	402	410	418	426	435	443

Source: Adapted from Clinical guidelines on the identification, evaluation, and treatment of overweight and obesity in adults: the evidence report. Retrieved June 2009 from www.nhlbi.nih.gov/guidelines/obesity/bmi_tbl.pdf.

Pain Assessment: The Fifth Vital Sign

PURPOSE

This chapter helps you learn the structure and function of pain pathways, understand the process of nociception, understand the rationale and methods of pain assessment, and accurately record the findings.

READING ASSIGNMENT

Jarvis: *Physical Examination and Health Assessment,* 6th ed., Chapter 10, pp. 159-174.

GLOSSARY

Study the following terms after completing the reading assignment. You should be able to cover the definition on the right and define the term out loud.

Acute pain . . . . short-term, self-limiting, often predictable trajectory; stops after injury heals

Breakthrough pain . . . . pain restarts or escalates before next scheduled analgesic dose

Chronic (persistent) pain . . . . . pain continues for 6 months or longer after initial injury

Cutaneous pain . . . . pain originating from skin surface or subcutaneous structures

Incident pain . . . . occurs predictably after specific movements

Modulation . . . . pain message is inhibited during this last phase of nociception

Neuropathic pain . . . . abnormal processing of pain message; burning, shooting in nature

Nociception . . . . process whereby noxious stimuli are perceived as pain; central and peripheral nervous systems are intact

Nociceptors . . . . specialized nerve endings that detect painful sensations

Pain . . . . "An unpleasant sensory and emotional experience associated with actual or potential tissue damage, or described in terms of such damage. Pain is always subjective" (American Pain Society).

Perception . . . . conscious awareness of painful sensation

Referred pain . . . . pain felt at a particular site but originates from another location

Somatic pain . . . . originating from muscle, bone, joints, tendons, or blood vessels

Transduction . . . . first phase of nociception whereby the painful stimulus is changed into an action potential

Transmission . . . . second phase of nociception whereby the pain impulse moves from the spinal cord to the brain

Visceral pain . . . . originating from interior organs such as the gallbladder or stomach

STUDY GUIDE

After completing the reading assignment, you should be able to answer the following questions in the spaces provided.

1. Describe the process of nociception using the four phases of:

    Transduction _____

    Transmission _____

    Perception _____

    Modulation _____

2. Identify the differences between nociceptive and neuropathic pain. What words will people use to describe nociceptive and neuropathic pain?

3. List various sources of pain.

4. Explain how acute and chronic pain differ in terms of nonverbal behaviors.

5. Identify the most reliable indicator of a person's pain.

6. Recall questions for an initial pain assessment.

7. Select pain assessment tools that are appropriate for adults, infants, and children.

8. Describe physical examination findings that may indicate pain.

9. Recall how poorly controlled acute and chronic pain adversely affect physiologic, social, and cognitive functioning.

CRITICAL THINKING QUESTIONS

1. What conditions are more likely to produce pain in the aging adult?

2. How would you modify your examination when the patient reports having abdominal pain?

3. How would you assess for pain in an individual with dementia?

4. What would you say to someone who tells you that infants do not remember pain and that they are too little for the pain to have any damaging effect?

5. What would you say to a colleague who remarks that the individual with Alzheimer disease does not feel pain and therefore does not require an analgesic?

Fill in the labels indicated on the following illustration.

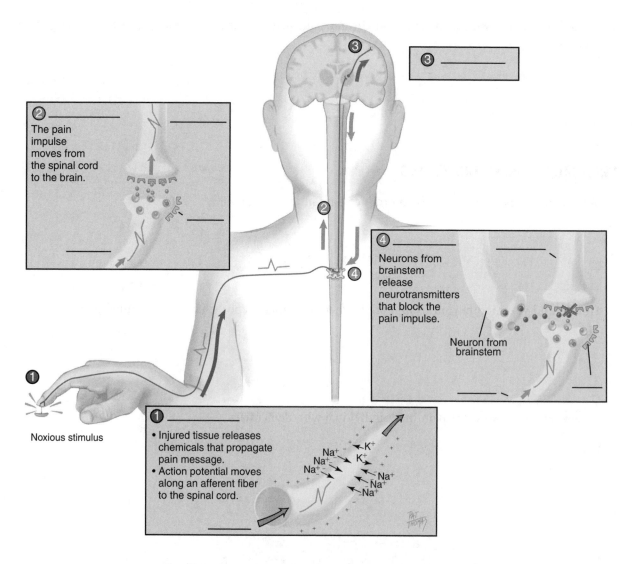

③ _____

② _____
The pain impulse moves from the spinal cord to the brain.

④ _____
Neurons from brainstem release neurotransmitters that block the pain impulse.

Neuron from brainstem

① _____
• Injured tissue releases chemicals that propagate pain message.
• Action potential moves along an afferent fiber to the spinal cord.

Na⁺ K⁺
Na⁺ K⁺
Na⁺
Na⁺
Na⁺
Na⁺

Noxious stimulus

REVIEW QUESTIONS

This test is for you to check your own mastery of the content. Answers are provided in Appendix A.

1. At what phase during nociception does the individual become aware of a painful sensation?

   a. modulation
   b. transduction
   c. perception
   d. transmission

2. While taking a history, the patient describes a burning, painful sensation that moves around his toes and bottoms of his feet. These symptoms are suggestive of:

   a. nociceptive pain.
   b. neuropathic pain.

3. During the physical examination, your patient is diaphoretic and pale and complains of pain directly over the LUQ of the abdomen. This would be categorized as:

   a. cutaneous pain.
   b. somatic pain.
   c. visceral pain.
   d. psychogenic pain.

4. While caring for a preterm infant, you are aware that:

   a. inhibitory neurotransmitters are in sufficient supply by 15 weeks' gestation.
   b. the fetus has less capacity to feel pain.
   c. repetitive blood draws have minimal long-term consequences.
   d. the preterm infant is more sensitive to painful stimuli.

5. The most reliable indicator of pain in the adult is:

   a. degree of physical functioning.
   b. nonverbal behaviors.
   c. MRI findings.
   d. the patient's self-report.

6. While examining a broken arm of a 4-year-old boy, select the appropriate assessment tool to evaluate his pain status.

   a. 0-10 numeric rating scale
   b. The Wong-Baker scale
   c. Simple descriptor scale
   d. 0-5 numeric rating scale

7. Normal age-related findings in the lower extremities of an 80-year-old woman would be:

   a. crepitus.
   b. joint swelling.
   c. diminished strength bilaterally.
   d. unilateral muscle atrophy.

8. When a person presents with acute pain of the abdomen, after the initial examination, it is best to withhold analgesic until diagnostic testing is completed and a diagnosis is made.

   a. True
   b. False

9. For older-adult postoperative patients, poorly controlled acute pain places them at higher risk for:

   a. atelectasis.
   b. increased myocardial oxygen demand.
   c. impaired wound healing.
   d. all of the above.

10. A 30-year-old female reports having persistent intense pain in her right arm related to trauma sustained from a car accident 5 months ago. She states that the slightest touch or clothing can exacerbate the pain. This report is suggestive of:

    a. referred pain.
    b. psychogenic pain.
    c. Complex Regional Pain I.
    d. cutaneous pain.

11. The CRIES is an appropriate pain assessment tool for:

    a. cognitively impaired older adults.
    b. children ages 2 to 8 years.
    c. infants.
    d. preterm and term neonates.

12. A pain problem should be anticipated in a cognitively impaired older adult with a history of:

    a. constipation.
    b. peripheral vascular disease.
    c. COPD.
    d. Parkinson disease.

13. Pain in the aging adult is considered to be:

    a. part of the normal degenerative process.
    b. perceived to a lesser degree.
    c. an expected finding.
    d. unrelated to the aging process.

14. A common physiologic change that occurs with pain is:

    a. polyuria.
    b. hyperventilation.
    c. hyperactive bowel sounds.
    d. tachycardia.

SKILLS LABORATORY/CLINICAL SETTING

You are now ready for the clinical component of the pain assessment. The purpose of the clinical component is to practice the examination on a peer in the skills laboratory or on a patient in the clinical setting and to achieve the following.

Clinical Objectives

1. Obtain an initial pain assessment on a classmate or patient.

2. Demonstrate a physical examination on a painful area, and identify abnormal findings.

3. Select appropriate pain assessment tools for further follow-up and monitoring.

4. Record the history and physical examination findings accurately, assess the nature of the pain, and develop an appropriate plan of care.

Nutritional Assessment

PURPOSE

This chapter helps you learn the components of nutritional assessment, including the assessment of dietary intake and nutritional status of individuals; identify the possible occurrence, nature, and extent of impaired nutritional status (ranging from undernutrition to overnutrition); and record the assessment accurately.

READING ASSIGNMENT

Jarvis: *Physical Examination and Health Assessment*, 6th ed., Chapter 11, pp. 175-202.

GLOSSARY

Study the following terms after completing the reading assignment. You should be able to cover the definition on the right and define the term out loud.

Android obesity . . . . excess body fat that is placed predominantly within the abdomen and upper body, as opposed to the hips and thighs

Anthropometry . . . . measurement of the body (e.g., height, weight, circumferences, skinfold thickness)

Body mass index . . . . weight in kilograms divided by height in meters squared (W/H^2); value of 30 or more is indicative of obesity; value of less than 18.5 is indicative of undernutrition

Diet history . . . . a detailed record of dietary intake obtainable from 24-hour recalls, food frequency questionnaires, food diaries, and similar methods

Gynoid obesity . . . . excess body fat that is placed predominantly within the hips and thighs

Kwashiorkor . . . . primarily a protein deficiency characterized by edema, growth failure, and muscle wasting

Malnutrition . . . . may mean any nutrition disorder but usually refers to long-term nutritional inadequacies or excesses

Marasmic kwashiorkor . . . . combination of chronic energy deficit and chronic or acute protein deficiency

Marasmus . . . . results from energy and protein deficiency, presenting with significant loss of body weight, skeletal muscle, and adipose tissue mass, but with serum protein concentrations relatively intact

Mid–arm muscle area (MAMA) . . . . a more sensitive indicator of lean body mass than MAC or MAMC

Mid–upper arm circumference (MAC) . . . . an indicator of lean body mass and fat stores

Mid–upper arm muscle circumference (MAMC) . . . . . . an indicator of lean body mass calculated from the triceps skinfold thickness and the mid–upper arm circumference

Nutritional monitoring . . . . . . assessment of dietary or nutritional status at intermittent times with the aim of detecting changes in the dietary or nutritional status of a population

Nutrition screening . . . . a process used to identify individuals at nutrition risk or with nutritional problems

Obesity . . . . excessive accumulation of body fat; usually defined as 20% above desirable weight or body mass index 30.0 to 39.9

Protein-calorie malnutrition (PCM) . . . . inadequate consumption of protein and energy, resulting in a gradual body wasting and increased susceptibility to infection

Recommended dietary allowance (RDA) . . . . levels of intake of essential nutrients considered to be adequate to meet the nutritional needs of practically all healthy persons

Serum proteins . . . . proteins present in serum that are indicators of the body's visceral protein status (e.g., albumin, prealbumin, transferrin)

Skinfold thickness . . . . double fold of skin and underlying subcutaneous tissue that is measured with skinfold calipers at various body sites

Waist-to-hip ratio (WHR) . . . . waist or abdominal circumference divided by the hip or gluteal circumference; method for assessing fat distribution

STUDY GUIDE

After completing the reading assignment, you should be able to answer the following questions in the spaces provided.

1. Define *nutritional status*.

2. Describe the unique nutritional needs for various developmental periods throughout the life cycle.

3. Describe the role cultural heritage and values may play in an individual's nutritional intake.

4. State 3 purposes of a nutritional assessment.

5. Describe 4 sources of error that may occur when using the 24-hour diet recall.

6. Explain the clinical changes associated with each type of malnutrition:

Obesity _____

Marasmus _____

Kwashiorkor _____

Marasmus/kwashiorkor mix _____

REVIEW QUESTIONS

This test is for you to check your own mastery of the content. Answers are provided in Appendix A.

1. The balance between nutrient intake and nutrient requirements is described as:

   a. undernutrition.
   b. malnutrition.
   c. nutritional status.
   d. overnutrition.

2. To support the synthesis of maternal and fetal tissue during pregnancy, a weight gain of _____ pounds is recommended.

   a. 25 to 35
   b. 28 to 40
   c. 15 to 25
   d. Recommendation depends on BMI of mother at the start of the pregnancy.

3. Which of the following are normal, expected changes with aging?

   a. increase in energy needs
   b. increase in body water
   c. decrease in height
   d. increase in AP diameter of the chest

4. Which of the following data would be obtained as part of a nutritional screening?

   a. temperature, pulse, and respiration
   b. blood pressure and genogram
   c. weight and nutrition intake history
   d. serum creatinine levels

5. Current dietary guidelines recommend that complex carbohydrates make up _____% of total calorie intake.

   a. 30
   b. 40
   c. 60
   d. 75

6. The 24-hour recall of dietary intake:

   a. is an anthropometric measure of calories consumed.
   b. is a questionnaire or interview of everything eaten within the last 24 hours.
   c. is the same as a food frequency questionnaire.
   d. is a form of food diary.

7. The nutritional needs of a patient with trauma or major surgery:

   a. are met by fat reserves in obese individuals.
   b. may be two to three times greater than normal.
   c. can be met with intravenous fluids, supplemented with vitamins and electrolytes.
   d. are met by glycogen reserves.

8. Mary, a 15-year-old, has come for a school physical. During the interview, the examiner is told that menarche has not occurred. An explanation to be explored is:

   a. nutritional deficiency.
   b. alcohol intake.
   c. smoking history.
   d. possible elevated blood sugar.

9. Older adults are at risk for alteration in nutritional status. From the individuals described below, select the individual(s) who appear(s) least at risk.

   a. an 80-year-old widow who lives alone
   b. a 65-year-old widower who visits a senior center with a meal program 5 days a week
   c. a 70-year-old with poor dentition who lives with a son
   d. a 73-year-old couple with low income and no transportation

10. Body weight as a percentage of ideal body weight is calculated to assess for malnutrition. Severe malnutrition is diagnosed when current body weight is:

    a. 80% to 90% of ideal weight.
    b. 70% to 80% of ideal weight.
    c. less than 70% of ideal body weight.
    d. 120% of ideal body weight.

11. The examiner is completing an initial assessment for a patient being admitted to a long-term care facility. The patient is unable to stand for a measurement of height. To obtain this important anthropometric information, the examiner may:

    a. measure the waist-to-hip circumference.
    b. estimate the body mass index.
    c. measure arm span.
    d. obtain a mid–upper arm muscle circumference to estimate skeletal muscle reserve.

12. Which assessment finding indicates nutrition risk?

    a. BMI = 24
    b. serum albumin = 2.5 g/dL
    c. current weight = 200 pounds
    d. BMI = 19

13. Marasmus is often characterized by:

    a. severely depleted visceral proteins.
    b. elevated triglycerides.
    c. hyperglycemia.
    d. low weight for height.

14. Which BMI category in adults is indicative of obesity?

    a. 18.5-24.9
    b. 25.0-29.9
    c. 30.0-39.9
    d. <18.5

15. When reviewing the laboratory report (shown below) of a patient, the examiner realizes this patient is demonstrating:

    a. no evidence of protein depletion.
    b. mild visceral protein deficiency based on the serum albumin.
    c. moderate protein depletion based on the serum transferrin.
    d. moderate protein loss based on the serum prealbumin.

Laboratory Report	
Serum albumin	4.0 g/dL
Serum transferrin	200 mg/dL
Serum prealbumin	9 mg/dL

16. Why should the examiner ask about the use of medications when assessing nutritional status?

    a. Medication allergies are on the rise and a major health concern.
    b. Many drugs can interact with nutrients and impair their digestion, absorption, metabolism, or utilization.
    c. Patients readily discuss their daily use of vitamin and mineral supplements when asked.
    d. The use of anabolic steroids can reduce muscle size and physical performance.

SKILLS LABORATORY/CLINICAL SETTING

You are now ready for the clinical component of the nutritional assessment. The purpose of the clinical component is to practice the steps of the assessment on a peer in the skills laboratory and to achieve the following.

Clinical Objectives

1. Identify persons at risk for developing malnutrition.

2. Develop an appreciation for cultural influences on nutritional status.

3. Use anthropometric measures and laboratory data to assess the nutritional status of an individual.

4. Use nutritional assessment in the provision of health care.

5. Record the assessment findings accurately.

Instructions

Gather nutritional assessment forms and anthropometric equipment. Practice the steps of the *Malnutrition Screening Tool* on a peer in the skills laboratory.

Next, practice the steps of the *Subjective Global Assessment Form* on a peer in the skills laboratory or on a patient in the clinical setting. This will give you practice with a more detailed history, collecting food intake measures, physical examination signs, and performing anthropometric measures.

Finally, review the questions in the *Mini Nutritional Assessment* with an aging adult. Persons identified as being at risk (MNA score 0-11 points) should undergo a more comprehensive assessment.

MALNUTRITION SCREENING TOOL (MST)

Have you lost weight recently without trying?
No	0
Unsure	2

If yes, how much weight (kilograms) have you lost?
1-5	1
6-10	2
11-15	3
>15	4
Unsure	2

Have you been eating poorly because of a decreased appetite?
No	0
Yes	1
Total	

Score of 2 or more = Patient at risk for malnutrition.

REGIONAL WRITE-UP—NUTRITIONAL ASSESSMENT

Date _____

Examiner _____

Patient _____ Age _____ Gender _____

Reason for visit _____

Features of the Scored Patient-Generated Subjective Global Assessment (PG-SGA)

(Select appropriate category with a checkmark, or enter numerical value where indicated by "#".)

A. History
1. Weight change
   Overall loss in past 6 months: amount = #_____ kg; % loss = #_____
   Change in past 2 weeks: _____ increase, _____ no change, _____ decrease
2. Dietary intake change (relative to normal)
   ____ No change
   ____ Change _____ duration = #_____ weeks
   ____ Type: _____ suboptimal solid diet _____ full liquid diet _____ hypocaloric liquids
   ____ starvation
3. Gastrointestinal symptoms (that persisted for >2 weeks)
   ____ none _____ nausea _____ vomiting
   ____ diarrhea _____ anorexia
4. Functional capacity
   ____ No dysfuncion (e.g., full capacity)
   ____ Dysfunction _____ duration = #_____ weeks
   ____ Type: _____ working suboptimally _____ ambulatory _____ bedridden
5. Disease and its relation to nutritional requirements
   Primary diagnosis (specify)
   Metabolic demand (stress): _____ no stress _____ low stress _____ moderate stress
   _____ high stress

B. Physical (FOR EACH TRAIT SPECIFY 0 = NORMAL, 1+ = MILD, 2+ = MODERATE, 3+ = SEVERE)

   #____ loss of subcutaneous fat (triceps, chest)

   #____ muscle wasting (quadriceps, deltoids)

   #____ ankle edema

   #____ sacral edema

   #____ ascites

C. SGA rating (SELECT ONE)
   ____ A = Well nourished
   ____ B = Moderately malnourished (or suspected of being malnourished)
   ____ C = Severely malnourished

Reprinted with permission from Detsky, A.J., McLaughlin, J.R., Baker, J.P., et al. (1987). What is subjective global assessment of nutritional status? *JPEN Journal of Parenteral and Enteral Nutrition, 11*, 9.

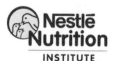

Mini Nutritional Assessment
MNA®

Last name:	First name:	Sex:	Date:

Age:	Weight, kg:	Height, cm:	I.D. number:

Complete the screen by filling in the boxes with the appropriate numbers. Total the numbers for the final screening score.

Screening

A Has food intake declined over the past 3 months due to loss of appetite, digestive problems, chewing or swallowing difficulties?

0 = severe decrease in food intake
1 = moderate decrease in food intake
2 = no decrease in food intake ☐

B Weight loss during the last 3 months

0 = weight loss greater than 3 kg (6.6 lbs)
1 = does not know
2 = weight loss between 1 and 3 kg (2.2 and 6.6 lbs)
3 = no weight loss ☐

C Mobility

0 = bed or chair bound
1 = able to get out of bed / chair but does not go out
2 = goes out ☐

D Has suffered psychological stress or acute disease in the past 3 months?

0 = yes 2 = no ☐

E Neuropsychological problems

0 = severe dementia or depression
1 = mild dementia
2 = no psychological problems ☐

F1 Body Mass Index (BMI) (weight in kg) / (height in m^2)

0 = BMI less than 19
1 = BMI 19 to less than 21
2 = BMI 21 to less than 23
3 = BMI 23 or greater ☐

IF BMI IS NOT AVAILABLE, REPLACE QUESTION F1 WITH QUESTION F2.
DO NOT ANSWER QUESTION F2 IF QUESTION F1 IS ALREADY COMPLETED.

F2 Calf circumference (CC) in cm

0 = CC less than 31
3 = CC 31 or greater ☐

Screening score
(max. 14 points) ☐☐

12-14 points: Normal nutritional status
8-11 points: At risk of malnutrition
0-7 points: Malnourished

For a more in-depth assessment, complete the full MNA® which is available at www.mna-elderly.com

Ref. Vellas B, Villars H, Abellan G, et al. *Overview of the MNA® - Its History and Challenges.* J Nutr Health Aging 2006;10:456-465.

Rubenstein LZ, Harker JO, Salva A, Guigoz Y, Vellas B. *Screening for Undernutrition in Geriatric Practice: Developing the Short-Form Mini Nutritional Assessment (MNA-SF).* J. Geront 2001;56A: M366-377.

Guigoz Y. *The Mini-Nutritional Assessment (MNA®) Review of the Literature - What does it tell us?* J Nutr Health Aging 2006; 10:466-487.

For more information: www.mna-elderly.com

CHAPTER
12

Skin, Hair, and Nails

PURPOSE

This chapter helps you learn the structure and function of the skin and its appendages; understand the rationale for and the methods of inspection and palpation of the skin; and record the assessment accurately.

READING ASSIGNMENT

Jarvis: *Physical Examination and Health Assessment*, 6th ed., Chapter 12, pp. 203-250.

GLOSSARY

Study the following terms after completing the reading assignment. You should be able to cover the definition on the right and define the term out loud.

Alopecia . . . . (baldness) hair loss

Annular . . . . circular shape to skin lesion

Bulla . . . . elevated cavity containing free fluid larger than 1 cm diameter

Confluent . . . . skin lesions that run together

Crust . . . . thick, dried-out exudate left on skin when vesicles/pustules burst or dry up

Cyanosis . . . . dusky blue color to skin or mucous membranes due to increased amount of unoxygenated hemoglobin

Erosion . . . . scooped out, shallow depression in skin

Erythema . . . . intense redness of the skin due to excess blood in dilated superficial capillaries, as in fever or inflammation

Excoriation . . . . self-inflicted abrasion on skin due to scratching

Fissure . . . . linear crack in skin extending into dermis

Furuncle . . . . (boil) suppurative inflammatory skin lesion due to infected hair follicle

Hemangioma . . . . skin lesion due to benign proliferation of blood vessels in the dermis

Iris . . . . target shape of skin lesion

Jaundice . . . . yellow color to skin, palate, and sclera due to excess bilirubin in the blood

Keloid . . . . hypertrophic scar, elevated beyond site of original injury

Lichenification . . . . tightly packed set of papules that thickens skin, from prolonged intense scratching

Lipoma . . . . benign fatty tumor

Maceration . . . . softening of tissue by soaking

Macule . . . . flat skin lesion with only a color change

Nevus . . . . (mole) circumscribed skin lesion due to excess melanocytes

Nodule . . . . elevated skin lesion, >1 cm diameter

Pallor . . . . excessively pale, whitish pink color to lightly pigmented skin

Papule . . . . palpable skin lesion, <1 cm diameter

Plaque . . . . skin lesion in which papules coalesce or come together

Pruritus . . . . itching

Purpura . . . . red-purple skin lesion due to blood in tissues from breaks in blood vessels

Pustule . . . . elevated cavity containing thick, turbid fluid

Scale . . . . compact desiccated flakes of skin from shedding of dead skin cells

Telangiectasia . . . . skin lesion due to permanently enlarged and dilated blood vessels that are visible

Ulcer . . . . sloughing of necrotic inflammatory tissue that causes a deep depression in skin, extending into dermis

Vesicle . . . . elevated cavity containing free fluid up to 1 cm diameter

Wheal . . . . raised red skin lesion due to interstitial fluid

Zosteriform . . . . linear shape of skin lesion along a nerve route

STUDY GUIDE

After completing the reading assignment, you should be able to answer the following questions in the spaces provided.

1. List the 3 layers associated with the skin, and describe the contents of each layer.

2. Define 2 types of human hair.

3. Differentiate between sebaceous, eccrine, and apocrine glands.

4. List at least 5 functions of the skin.

5. List at least 6 variables that are external to the skin itself that can influence skin color.

6. Describe the appearance of pallor, erythema, cyanosis, and jaundice, both in light-skinned and in dark-skinned persons. State common causes of each.

7. List causes of changes in skin temperature, texture, moisture, mobility, and turgor.

8. Describe each grade on the 4-point grading scale for pitting edema.

9. Distinguish the terms *primary* versus *secondary* in reference to skin lesions.

10. The white linear markings that normally are visible through the nail and on the pink nail bed are termed _____.

11. Describe the following findings that are common variations on the infant's skin:

    Mongolian spot _____

    Café au lait spot _____

    Erythema toxicum _____

    Cutis marmorata _____

    Physiologic jaundice _____

    Milia _____

12. Describe the following findings that are common variations on the aging adult's skin:

    Lentigines _____

    Seborrheic keratosis _____

    Actinic keratosis _____

    Acrochordons (skin tags) _____

    Sebaceous hyperplasia _____

13. Differentiate between these purpuric lesions: petechiae; bruise; hematoma.

14. Differentiate between the appearance of the skin rash of these childhood illnesses: measles (rubeola); German measles (rubella); chickenpox (varicella).

15. List and describe the 4 stages of pressure ulcer development.

16. Contrast a furuncle with an abscess.

17. Describe the appearance of these conditions of the nails: koilonychia; paronychia; Beau's line; splinter hemorrhages; onycholysis; clubbing.

18. Define and give an example of the following primary skin lesions: macule; papule; plaque; nodule; tumor; wheal; vesicle; pustule.

    And of these secondary lesions: crust; scale; fissure; erosion; ulcer.

Fill in the labels indicated on the following illustrations.

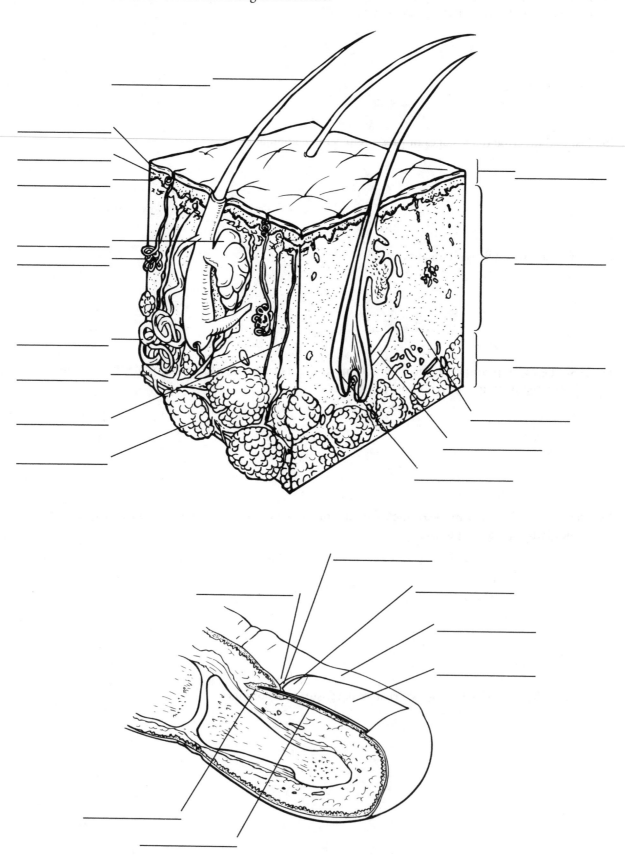

REVIEW QUESTIONS

This test is for you to check your own mastery of the content. Answers are provided in Appendix A.

1. Select the best description of the secretion of the eccrine glands.

   a. thick, milky
   b. dilute saline solution
   c. protective lipid substance
   d. keratin

2. Nevus is the medical term for:

   a. a freckle.
   b. a birthmark.
   c. an infected hair follicle.
   d. a mole.

3. To assess for early jaundice, you will assess:

   a. sclera and hard palate.
   b. nail beds.
   c. lips.
   d. all visible skin surfaces.

4. Checking for skin temperature is best accomplished by using:

   a. palmar surface of the hands.
   b. ventral surface of the hands.
   c. fingertips.
   d. dorsal surface of the hands.

5. Skin turgor is assessed by picking up a large fold of skin on the anterior chest under the clavicle. This is done to determine the presence of:

   a. edema.
   b. dehydration.
   c. vitiligo.
   d. scleroderma.

6. You note a lesion during an examination. Select the description that is most complete.

   a. raised, irregular lesion the size of a quarter, located on dorsum of left hand
   b. open lesion with no drainage or odor, approximately ¼ inch in diameter
   c. pedunculated lesion below left scapula with consistent red color, no drainage or odor
   d. dark brown, raised lesion, with irregular border, on dorsum of right foot, 3 cm in size with no drainage

7. You examine nail beds for clubbing. The normal angle between the nail base and the nails is:

   a. 60 degrees.
   b. 100 degrees.
   c. 160 degrees.
   d. 180 degrees.

8. The capillary beds should refill after being depressed in:

   a. <1 second.
   b. >2 seconds.
   c. 1-2 seconds.
   d. time is not significant as long as color returns.

9. During a routine visit, M.B., age 78, asks about small, round, flat, brown macules on the hands. Your best response after examining the areas is:

   a. "These are the result of sun exposure and do not require treatment."
   b. "These are related to exposure to the sun. They may become cancerous."
   c. "These are the skin tags that occur with aging. No treatment is required."
   d. "I'm glad you brought this to my attention. I will arrange for a biopsy."

Jarvis, Carolyn: PHYSICAL EXAMINATION AND HEALTH ASSESSMENT: Sixth Edition,
Student Laboratory Manual. Copyright © 2012, 2008, 2004, 2000, 1996 by Saunders, an imprint of Elsevier Inc. All rights reserved.

10. An area of thin, shiny skin with decreased visibility of normal skin markings is called:

    a. lichenification.
    b. plaque.
    c. atrophy.
    d. keloid.

11. Flattening of the angle between the nail and its base is:

    a. found in subacute bacterial endocarditis.
    b. a description of spoon-shaped nails.
    c. related to calcium deficiency.
    d. described as clubbing.

12. The configuration for individual lesions arranged in circles or arcs, as occurs with ringworm, is called:

    a. linear.
    b. clustered.
    c. annular.
    d. gyrate.

13. The "A" in the ABCDE rule stands for:

    a. accuracy.
    b. appearance.
    c. asymmetry.
    d. attenuated.

14. A risk factor for melanoma is:

    a. brown eyes.
    b. darkly pigmented skin.
    c. skin that freckles or burns before tanning.
    d. use of sunscreen products.

15. Lyme disease is more prevalent:

    a. from May through September.
    b. along the West Coast.
    c. in children younger than 3 years.
    d. in those participating in water sports.

16. Herpes zoster (shingles):

    a. caused by bacteria.
    b. lesion on only one side of body; does not cross midline.
    c. has absence of pain or edema.
    d. forms pustular, umbilicated lesions.

17. Clubbing can be assessed by:

    a. observing for transverse ridges in the nails.
    b. the presence of pits in the nails.
    c. noting a change in the angle of the nail base.
    d. palpating a rigid nail base.

18. Milia occur because:

    a. sebum occludes skin follicles.
    b. of a vascular occlusion in the skin.
    c. excess carotene is ingested.
    d. of a genetic variation in skin tone.

Match column A to column B—items in column B may be used more than once.

Column A—Descriptor

19. _____ basal cell layer

20. _____ aids protection by cushioning

21. _____ collagen

22. _____ adipose tissue

23. _____ uniformly thin

24. _____ stratum corneum

25. _____ elastic tissue

Column B—Skin layer

a. epidermis

b. dermis

c. subcutaneous layer

Column A—Descriptor

26. _____ pallor

27. _____ erythema

28. _____ cyanosis

29. _____ jaundice

Column B—Color change

a. intense redness of the skin due to excess blood in the dilated superficial capillaries

b. bluish mottled color that signifies decreased perfusion

c. absence of red-pink tones from the oxygenated hemoglobin in blood

d. increase in bilirubin in the blood causing a yellow color in the skin

Column A—Descriptor

30. _____ tiny, punctate red macules and papules on the cheeks, trunk, chest, back, and buttocks

31. _____ lower half of body turns red, upper half blanches

32. _____ transient mottling on trunk and extremities

33. _____ bluish color around the lips, hands, fingernails, feet, and toenails

34. _____ large round or oval patch of light brown usually present at birth

35. _____ yellowing of skin, sclera, and mucous membranes due to increased numbers of red blood cells hemolyzed following birth

36. _____ yellow-orange color in light-skinned persons from large amounts of foods containing carotene

Column B—Skin color change

a. harlequin

b. erythema toxicum

c. acrocyanosis

d. physiologic jaundice

e. carotenemia

f. café au lait

g. cutis marmorata

SKILLS LABORATORY/CLINICAL SETTING

You are now ready for the clinical component of the integumentary system. Usually the clinical examination of the integumentary system is performed along with the examination of each particular body region. The purpose of practicing the steps of this examination separately is so that you begin to think of the skin and its appendages as a separate organ system and so that you learn the components of skin examination.

Clinical Objectives

1. Inspect and palpate the skin, noting its color, vascularity, edema, moisture, temperature, texture, thickness, mobility, turgor, and any lesions.

2. Inspect the fingernails, noting color, shape, and any lesions.

3. Inspect the hair, noting texture, distribution, and any lesions.

4. Record the history and physical examination findings accurately, reach an assessment of the health state, and develop a plan of care.

Instructions

Prepare the examination setting. Wash your hands. Practice the steps of the examination on a peer in the skills laboratory, giving appropriate instructions as you proceed. Choosing a peer from an ethnic background other than your own will further heighten your recognition of the range of normal skin tones. Record your findings using the regional write-up sheet that follows. The front of the page is intended as a worksheet; the back of the page is intended for your narrative summary recording using the SOAP format.

Note the student performance checklist that follows the regional write-up sheet. It lists the essential behaviors you should display as an examiner, and it may be used by your clinical instructor to evaluate your clinical teaching of the skin self-examination.

NOTES

REGIONAL WRITE-UP—SKIN, HAIR, AND NAILS

Date _____

Examiner _____

Patient _____ Age _____ Gender _____

Reason for visit _____

I. Health History

	No	Yes, explain
1. Any past **skin disease?**		
2. Any change in skin color or **pigmentation?**		
3. Any changes in a **mole?**		
4. Excessive **dryness** or **moisture?**		
5. Any skin **itching?**		
6. Any excess **bruising?**		
7. Any skin **rash** or **lesions?**		
8. Taking any **medications?**		
9. Any recent hair loss?		
10. Any change in nails?		
11. Any environmental hazards for skin?		
12. How do you take care of skin? Sunscreen?		

II. Physical Examination

A. Inspect and palpate skin

Color _____

Pigmentation _____

Temperature _____

Moisture _____

Texture _____

Thickness _____

Any edema _____

Mobility and turgor _____

Vascularity and bruising _____

Any lesions (describe) _____

B. Inspect and palpate hair

Color _____

Texture _____

Distribution _____

Any lesions (describe) _____

C. Inspect and palpate nails

Shape and contour _____

Consistency _____

Distribution _____

Color _____

Capillary refill _____

D. Teach skin self-examination

REGIONAL WRITE-UP—SKIN, HAIR, AND NAILS

Summarize your findings using the SOAP format.

Subjective (Reason for seeking care, health history)

Objective (Physical examination findings)   Record distribution of any rash or lesions below

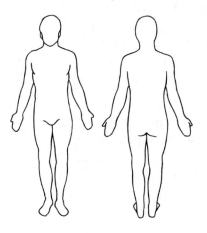

Assessment (Assessment of problem, diagnosis)

Plan (Diagnostic evaluation, follow-up care, teaching)

STUDENT COMPETENCY CHECKLIST

TEACHING SKIN SELF-EXAMINATION (SSE)

	S	U	Comments
I. Cognitive			
A. Explain:			
1. Why skin is examined			
2. Who should perform skin self-examination			
3. Frequency of skin examination			
B. Define the ABCDE rule			
C. Describe any equipment the patient may need			
II. Performance			
A. Explains to patient need for SSE			
B. Instructs patient on technique of SSE by:			
1. demonstrating the order and body positioning for inspecting skin			
2. describing normal skin characteristics			
3. describing abnormal findings to look for			
C. Instructs patient to report unusual findings to nurse or physician at once			

NOTES

Head, Face, and Neck, Including Regional Lymphatics

PURPOSE

This chapter helps you learn the location and function of structures in the head and neck; learn to perform inspection and palpation of the head and neck; and record the assessment accurately.

READING ASSIGNMENT

Jarvis: *Physical Examination and Health Assessment*, 6th ed., Chapter 13, pp. 251-278.

MEDIA ASSIGNMENT

Jarvis: *Physical Examination and Health Assessment* DVD Series: Head, Eyes, and Ears.

GLOSSARY

Study the following terms after completing the reading assignment. You should be able to cover the definition on the right and define the term out loud.

Bruit . . . . blowing, swooshing sound heard through the stethoscope over an area of abnormal blood flow

Dysphagia . . . . difficulty in swallowing

Goiter . . . . increase in size of thyroid gland that occurs with hyperthyroidism

Lymphadenopathy . . . . enlargement of the lymph nodes due to infection, allergy, or neoplasm

Macrocephalic . . . . abnormally large head

Microcephalic . . . . abnormally small head

Normocephalic . . . . round symmetric skull that is appropriately related to body size

Torticollis . . . . head tilt due to shortening or spasm of one sternomastoid muscle

Vertigo . . . . illusory sensation of either the room or one's own body spinning; it is not the same as dizziness

STUDY GUIDE

After completing the reading assignment and the media assignment, you should be able to answer the following questions in the spaces provided.

1. The major neck muscles are the _____.

2. Name the borders of two regions in the neck—the anterior triangle and the posterior triangle.

3. List the facial structures that should appear symmetric when inspecting the head.

4. Describe the characteristics of lymph nodes often associated with:

   Acute infection _____

   Chronic inflammation _____

   Cancer _____

5. Differentiate *caput succedaneum* from *cephalhematoma* in the newborn infant.

6. Describe the tonic neck reflex in the infant.

7. Describe the characteristics of normal cervical lymph nodes during childhood.

8. List the condition(s) associated with parotid gland enlargement.

9. Describe the facial characteristics that occur with Down syndrome.

10. Contrast the facial characteristics of hyperthyroidism versus hypothyroidism.

Fill in the labels indicated on the following illustrations.

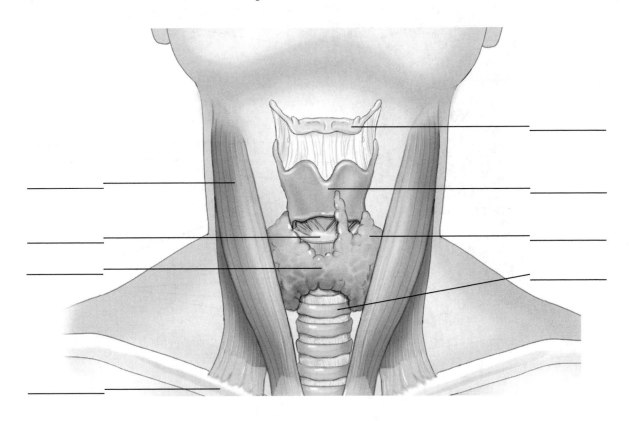

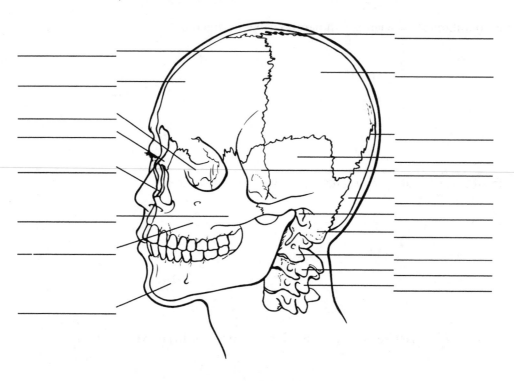

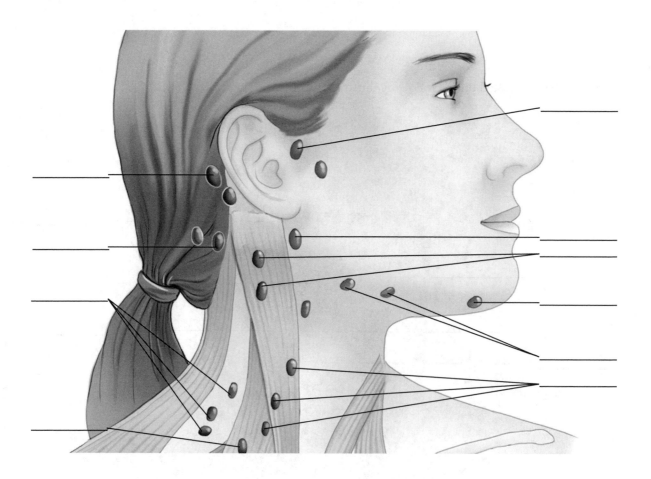

REVIEW QUESTIONS

This test is for you to check your own mastery of the content. Answers are provided in Appendix A.

1. Identify the facial bone that articulates at a joint instead of a suture.

   a. zygomatic
   b. maxilla
   c. nasal
   d. mandible

2. Identify the blood vessel that runs diagonally across the sternomastoid muscle.

   a. temporal artery
   b. carotid artery
   c. external jugular vein
   d. internal jugular vein

3. The isthmus of the thyroid gland lies just below the:

   a. mandible.
   b. cricoid cartilage.
   c. hyoid cartilage.
   d. thyroid cartilage.

4. Select the statement that is true regarding cluster headaches.

   a. may be precipitated by alcohol and daytime napping
   b. usual occurrence is two per month, each lasting 1 to 3 days
   c. characterized as throbbing
   d. tend to be supraorbital, retro-orbital, or frontotemporal

5. Select the symptom that is least likely to indicate a possible malignancy.

   a. history of radiation therapy to head, neck, or upper chest
   b. history of using chewing tobacco
   c. history of large alcohol consumption
   d. tenderness

6. Providing resistance while the patient shrugs the shoulders is a test of the status of cranial nerve:

   a. II.
   b. V.
   c. IX.
   d. XI.

7. Upon examination, the fontanels should feel:

   a. tense or bulging.
   b. depressed or sunken.
   c. firm, slightly concave, and well defined.
   d. pulsating.

8. If the thyroid gland is enlarged bilaterally, which of the following maneuvers is appropriate?

   a. Check for deviation of the trachea.
   b. Listen for a bruit over the carotid arteries.
   c. Listen for a murmur over the aortic area.
   d. Listen for a bruit over the thyroid lobes.

9. It is normal to palpate a few lymph nodes in the neck of a healthy person. What are the characteristics of these nodes?

   a. mobile, soft, nontender
   b. large, clumped, tender
   c. matted, fixed, tender, hard
   d. matted, fixed, nontender

10. Cephalhematoma is associated with:

   a. subperiosteal hemorrhage.
   b. increased intracranial pressure.
   c. Down syndrome.
   d. mental retardation.

11. Normal cervical lymph nodes are:

    a. smaller than 1 cm.
    b. warm to palpation.
    c. fixed.
    d. firm.

12. A throbbing, unilateral pain associated with nausea, vomiting, and photophobia is characteristic of:

    a. cluster headache.
    b. subarachnoid hemorrhage.
    c. migraine headache.
    d. tension headache.

13. Bell's palsy is characterized by:

    a. unilateral paralysis of half of the face.
    b. bulging eyeballs.
    c. a face that appears masklike.
    d. a puffy, edematous face.

14. The examiner suspects an infant's head is of abnormal size and can use which procedure to verify these findings?

    a. palpation
    b. measuring tape
    c. observing for symmetry of facial features
    d. noting absence of the tonic neck reflex

Match column A to column B.

Column A—Lymph nodes

15. _____ Preauricular

16. _____ Posterior auricular

17. _____ Occipital

18. _____ Submental

19. _____ Submandibular

20. _____ Jugulodigastric

21. _____ Superficial cervical

22. _____ Deep cervical

23. _____ Posterior cervical

24. _____ Supraclavicular

Column B—Location

a. above and behind the clavicle

b. deep under the sternomastoid muscle

c. in front of the ear

d. in the posterior triangle along the edge of the trapezius muscle

e. superficial to the mastoid process

f. at the base of the skull

g. halfway between the angle and the tip of the mandible

h. behind the tip of the mandible

i. under the angle of the mandible

j. overlying the sternomastoid muscle

SKILLS LABORATORY/CLINICAL SETTINGS

You are now ready for the clinical component of the head, face, and neck chapter. The purpose of the clinical component is to practice the steps of the head, face, and neck examination on a peer in the skills laboratory and to achieve the following objectives.

Clinical Objectives

1. Collect a health history related to pertinent signs and symptoms of the head and neck.

2. Inspect and palpate the skull noting size, contour, lumps, or tenderness.

3. Inspect the face noting facial expression, symmetry, skin characteristics, or lesions.

4. Inspect and palpate the neck for symmetry, range of motion, and integrity of lymph nodes, trachea, and thyroid gland.

5. Record the findings systematically, reach an assessment of the health state, and develop a plan of care.

Instructions

Prepare the examination setting. Wash your hands. Practice the steps of the examination on a peer in the skills laboratory, giving appropriate instructions as you proceed. Record your findings using the regional write-up sheet that follows. The front of the page is intended as a worksheet; the back of the page is intended for your narrative summary recording using the SOAP format.

NOTES

NOTES

REGIONAL WRITE-UP—HEAD, FACE, AND NECK

Date _____

Examiner _____

Patient _____ Age _____ Gender _____

Reason for visit _____

I. **Health History**

	No	Yes, explain

1. Any unusually frequent or unusually
    severe **headaches**?
2. Any **head injury**?
3. Experienced any **dizziness**?
4. Any neck **pain**?
5. Any **lumps** or **swelling** in head or neck?
6. Any surgery on head or neck?

II. **Physical Examination**
    A. **Inspect and palpate the skull**
        General size and contour _____
        Deformities, lumps, tenderness _____
        Temporal artery _____
        Temporomandibular joint _____
    B. **Inspect the face**
        Facial expression _____
        Symmetry of structures _____
        Involuntary movements _____
        Edema _____
        Masses or lesions _____
        Color and texture of skin _____
    C. **Inspect the neck**
        Symmetry _____
        Range of motion, active _____
        Test strength of cervical muscles _____
        Abnormal pulsations _____
        Enlargement of thyroid _____
        Enlargement of lymph and salivary glands _____
    D. **Palpate the lymph nodes**
        Exact location _____
        Size and shape _____
        Presence or absence of tenderness _____
        Freely movable, adherent to deeper structures, or matted together _____
        Presence of surrounding inflammation _____
        Texture (hard, soft, firm) _____
    E. **Palpate the trachea**
    F. **Palpate the thyroid gland**
    G. **Auscultate the thyroid gland (if enlarged)**

REGIONAL WRITE-UP—HEAD, FACE, AND NECK

Summarize your findings using the SOAP format.

Subjective (Reason for seeking care, health history)

Objective (Physical examination findings)

Assessment (Assessment of health state or problem, diagnosis)

Plan (Diagnostic evaluation, follow-up care, patient teaching)

PURPOSE

This chapter helps you learn the structure and function of the external and internal components of the eyes; learn the methods of examination of vision, external eye, and ocular fundus; and record the assessment accurately.

READING ASSIGNMENT

Jarvis: *Physical Examination and Health Assessment*, 6th ed., Chapter 14, pp. 279-322.

MEDIA ASSIGNMENT

Jarvis: *Physical Examination and Health Assessment* DVD Series: Head, Eyes, and Ears.

GLOSSARY

Study the following terms after completing the reading assignment. You should be able to cover the definition on the right and define the term out loud.

Accommodation............adaptation of the eye for near vision by increasing the curvature of the lens

Anisocoria.................unequal pupil size

Arcus senilis..............gray-white arc or circle around the limbus of the iris that is common with aging

Argyll Robertson pupil......pupil does not react to light; does constrict with accommodation

Astigmatism..............refractive error of vision due to differences in curvature in refractive surfaces of the eye (cornea and lens)

A-V crossing..............crossing paths of an artery and vein in the ocular fundus

Bitemporal hemianopsia.....loss of both temporal visual fields

Blepharitis...............inflammation of the glands and eyelash follicles along the margin of the eyelids

Cataract . . . . opacity of the lens of the eye that develops slowly with aging and gradually obstructs vision

Chalazion . . . . infection or retention cyst of a meibomian gland, showing as a beady nodule on the eyelid

Conjunctivitis . . . . infection of the conjunctiva, "pinkeye"

Cotton-wool area . . . . abnormal soft exudates visible as gray-white areas on the ocular fundus

Cup-disc ratio . . . . ratio of the width of the physiologic cup to the width of the optic disc, normally half or less

Diopter . . . . unit of strength of the lens settings on the ophthalmoscope that changes focus on the eye structures

Diplopia . . . . double vision

Drusen . . . . benign deposits on the ocular fundus that show as round yellow dots and occur commonly with aging

Ectropion . . . . lower eyelid loose and rolling outward

Entropion . . . . lower eyelid rolling inward

Exophthalmos . . . . protruding eyeballs

Fovea . . . . area of keenest vision at the center of the macula on the ocular fundus

Glaucoma . . . . a group of eye diseases characterized by increased intraocular pressure

Hordeolum . . . . (stye) red, painful pustule that is a localized infection of hair follicle at eyelid margin

Lid lag . . . . the abnormal white rim of sclera visible between the upper eyelid and the iris when a person moves the eyes downward

Macula . . . . round, darker area of the ocular fundus that mediates vision only from the central visual field

Microaneurysm . . . . abnormal finding of round red dots on the ocular fundus that are localized dilations of small vessels

Miosis . . . . constricted pupils

Mydriasis . . . . dilated pupils

Myopia . . . . "nearsighted"; refractive error in which near vision is better than far vision

Nystagmus . . . . involuntary, rapid, rhythmic movement of the eyeball

OD . . . . oculus dexter, or right eye

Optic atrophy . . . . pallor of the optic disc due to partial or complete death of optic nerve

Optic disc . . . . area of ocular fundus in which blood vessels exit and enter

OS . . . . oculus sinister, or left eye

Papilledema . . . . stasis of blood flow out of the ocular fundus; sign of increased intracranial pressure

Presbyopia . . . . decrease in power of accommodation that occurs with aging

Pterygium . . . . triangular opaque tissue on the nasal side of the conjunctiva that grows toward the center of the cornea

Ptosis . . . . drooping of upper eyelid over the iris and possibly covering pupil

Red reflex . . . . red glow that appears to fill the person's pupil when first visualized through the ophthalmoscope

Strabismus . . . . (squint, crossed eye) disparity of the eye axes

Xanthelasma. . . . . soft, raised yellow plaques occurring on the skin at the inner corners of the eyes

STUDY GUIDE

After completing the reading assignment and the media assignment, you should be able to answer the following questions in the spaces provided.

1. Name the 6 sets of extraocular muscles and the cranial nerve that innervates each one.

2. Name and describe the 3 concentric coats of the eyeball.

3. Name the functions of the ciliary body, the pupil, and the iris.

4. Describe the anterior chamber, the posterior chamber, and the vitreous body.

5. Describe how an image formed on the retina compares with its actual appearance in the outside world.

6. Describe the lacrimal system.

7. Define pupillary light reflex, fixation, and accommodation.

8. Concerning the pupillary light reflex, describe and contrast a direct light reflex with a consensual light reflex.

9. Identify common age-related changes in the eye.

10. Discuss the most common causes of decreased visual function in the older adult.

11. Explain the statement that normal visual acuity is 20/20.

12. Describe the method of testing for presbyopia.

13. To test for accommodation, the person focuses on a distant object and then shifts the gaze to a near object about 6 inches away. At near distance, you would expect the pupils to _____ (dilate/constrict), and the axes of the eyes to _____.

14. Concerning malalignment of the eye axes, contrast *phoria* with *tropia.*

15. Describe abnormal findings of tissue color that are possible on the conjunctiva and sclera, and describe their significance.

16. Describe the method of everting the upper eyelid for examination.

17. Contrast *pinguecula* with *pterygium.*

18. Contrast the use of the negative diopter or red lens settings with the positive diopter or black lens settings on the ophthalmoscope.

19. Explain the rationale for testing for strabismus during early childhood.

20. Describe these findings, and explain their significance: epicanthal fold; pseudostrabismus; ophthalmia neonatorum; Brushfield's spots.

21. Describe the following 4 types of "red eye," and explain their significance:

    a. Conjunctivitis:

    b. Subconjunctival hemorrhage:

    c. Iritis:

    d. Acute glaucoma:

Fill in the labels indicated on the following illustrations.

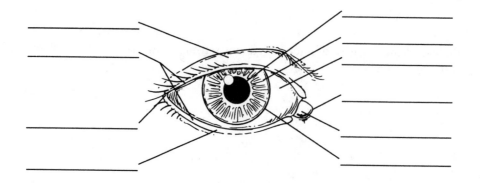

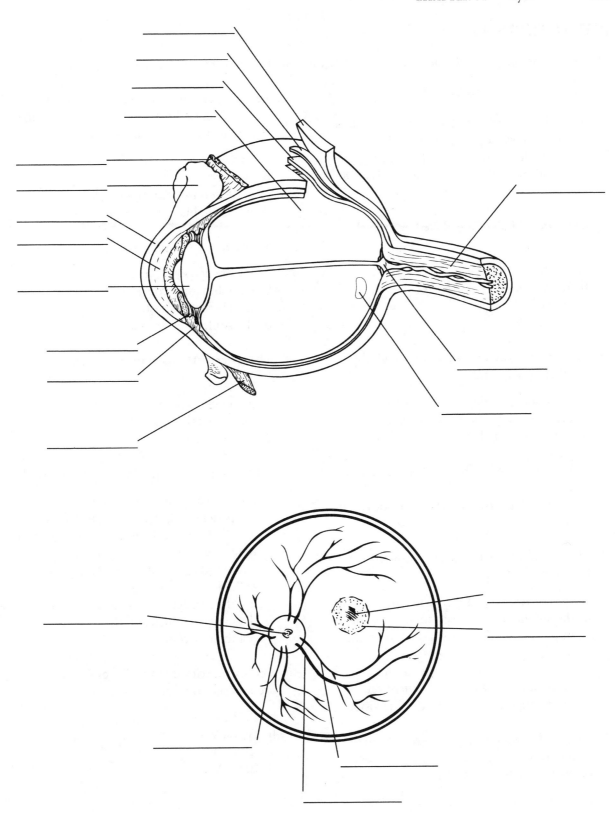

REVIEW QUESTIONS

This test is for you to check your own mastery of the content. Answers are provided in Appendix A.

1. The palpebral fissure is:

   a. the border between the cornea and sclera.
   b. the open space between the eyelids.
   c. the angle where the eyelids meet.
   d. visible on the upper and lower lids at the inner canthus.

2. The corneal reflex is mediated by cranial nerves:

   a. II and III.
   b. II and VI.
   c. V and VII.
   d. VI and IV.

3. The retinal structures viewed through the ophthalmoscope are:

   a. the optic disc, the retinal vessels, the general background, and the macula.
   b. the cornea, the lens, the choroid, and the ciliary body.
   c. the optic papilla, the sclera, the retina, and the iris.
   d. the pupil, the sclera, the ciliary body, and the macula.

4. The examiner records "positive consensual light reflex." This is:

   a. the convergence of the axes of the eyeballs.
   b. the simultaneous constriction of the other pupil when one eye is exposed to bright light.
   c. a reflex direction of the eye toward an object attracting a person's attention.
   d. the adaptation of the eye for near vision.

5. Several changes occur in the eye with the aging process. The thickening and yellowing of the lens is referred to as:

   a. presbyopia.
   b. floaters.
   c. macular degeneration.
   d. senile cataract.

6. Be alert to symptoms that may constitute an eye emergency. Identify the symptom(s) that should be referred immediately.

   a. floaters
   b. epiphora
   c. sudden onset of vision change
   d. photophobia

7. Visual acuity is assessed with:

   a. the Snellen eye chart.
   b. an ophthalmoscope.
   c. the Hirschberg test.
   d. the confrontation test.

8. The cover test is used to assess for:

   a. nystagmus.
   b. peripheral vision.
   c. muscle weakness.
   d. visual acuity.

9. When using the ophthalmoscope, you would:

   a. remove your own glasses and approach the patient's left eye with your left eye.
   b. leave light on in the examining room and remove glasses from the patient.
   c. remove glasses and set the diopter setting at 0.
   d. use the smaller white light and instruct the patient to focus on the ophthalmoscope.

10. The six muscles that control eye movement are innervated by cranial nerves:

    a. II, III, V.
    b. IV, VI, VII.
    c. III, IV, VI.
    d. II, III, VI.

11. Conjunctivitis is always associated with:

    a. absent red reflex.
    b. reddened conjunctiva.
    c. impairment of vision.
    d. fever.

12. A patient has blurred peripheral vision. You suspect glaucoma, and test the visual fields. A person with normal vision would see your moving finger temporally at:

    a. 50 degrees.
    b. 60 degrees.
    c. 90 degrees.
    d. 180 degrees.

13. A person is known to be blind in the left eye. What happens to the pupils when the right eye is illuminated by a penlight beam?

    a. No response in both.
    b. Both pupils constrict.
    c. Right pupil constricts, left has no response.
    d. Left pupil constricts, right has no response.

14. Use of the ophthalmoscope: an interruption of the red reflex occurs when:

    a. there is an opacity in the cornea or lens.
    b. the patient has pathology of the optic tract.
    c. the blood vessels are tortuous.
    d. the pupils are constricted.

15. One cause of visual impairment in aging adults is:

    a. strabismus.
    b. glaucoma.
    c. amblyopia.
    d. retinoblastoma.

16. Briefly describe the method of assessing the six cardinal fields of vision.

17. Documentation of an eye examination can include the term *PERRLA*. What does this mean?

    a. P—
    b. E—
    c. R—
    d. R—
    e. L—
    f. A—

18. What is the cause of the red reflex?

    a. petechial hemorrhages in the sclera
    b. diabetic retinopathy
    c. light reflecting from the retina
    d. blood in the vitreous

SKILLS LABORATORY/CLINICAL SETTING

You are now ready for the clinical component of the eye examination. The purpose of the clinical component is to practice the steps of the examination on a peer in the skills laboratory. Note that the first practice session usually takes a long time because there are so many separate steps. Be aware that success with the use of the ophthalmoscope is hard to achieve during the first practice session. Make sure you are holding the instrument correctly and practice focusing on various objects about the room before you try to look at a person's fundus. When you do examine a peer's eye, make sure to offer occasional rest times. It is very tiring for the "patient" to have the ophthalmoscope light shining in the eye. During the first practice session, aim for finding the red reflex and a retinal vessel or two; if you can locate the optic disc, so much the better.

Clinical Objectives

1. Collect a health history related to pertinent signs and symptoms of the eye system.

2. Demonstrate and explain assessment of visual acuity, visual fields, external eye structures, and ocular fundus.

3. Record the history and physical examination findings accurately, reach an assessment of the health state, and develop a plan of care.

Instructions

Prepare the examination setting. Wash your hands. Practice the steps of the examination on a peer in the skills laboratory, giving appropriate instructions as you proceed. Record your findings using the regional write-up sheet that follows. The front of the page is intended as a worksheet; the back of the page is intended for your narrative summary recording using the SOAP format.

NOTES

REGIONAL WRITE-UP—EYES

Date _____

Examiner _____

Patient _____ Age _____ Gender _____

Reason for visit _____

I. **Health History**

	No	Yes, explain
1. Any **difficulty seeing** or blurring?	_____	_____
2. Any eye **pain**?	_____	_____
3. Any history of **crossed eyes**?	_____	_____
4. Any **redness** or **swelling** in eyes?	_____	_____
5. Any **watering** or **tearing**?	_____	_____
6. Any **injury** or **surgery** to eye?	_____	_____
7. Ever tested for **glaucoma**?	_____	_____
8. Wear **glasses** or **contact lenses**?	_____	_____
9. Ever had vision tested?	_____	_____
10. Taking any medications?	_____	_____

II. **Physical Examination**
  A. **Test visual acuity**
    Snellen eye chart _____
    Pocket vision screener for near vision _____
  B. **Test visual fields**
    Confrontation test _____
  C. **Inspect extraocular muscle function**
    Corneal light reflex _____
    Cover test _____
    Diagnostic positions test _____
  D. **Inspect external eye structures**
    General _____
    Eyebrows _____
    Eyelids and lashes _____
    Eyeballs _____
    Conjunctiva and sclera _____
    Lacrimal gland, puncta _____
  E. **Inspect anterior eyeball structures**
    Cornea _____
    Iris _____
    Pupil size _____
    Pupil direct and consensual light reflex _____
    Accommodation _____
  F. **Inspect ocular fundus**
    Optic disc _____
    Vessels _____
    General background of fundus _____
    Macula _____

REGIONAL WRITE-UP—EYES

Summarize your findings using the SOAP format.

Subjective (Reason for seeking care, health history)

Objective (Physical examination findings)

Record findings on diagram below

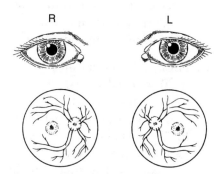

Assessment (Assessment of problem, diagnosis)

Plan (Diagnostic evaluation, follow-up care, teaching)

PURPOSE

This chapter helps you learn the structure and function of the ears; learn the methods of examination of hearing, external ear structures, and tympanic membrane using the otoscope; and record the assessment accurately.

READING ASSIGNMENT

Jarvis: *Physical Examination and Health Assessment*, 6th ed., Chapter 15, pp. 323-350.

MEDIA ASSIGNMENT

Jarvis: *Physical Examination and Health Assessment* DVD Series: Head, Eyes, and Ears.

GLOSSARY

Study the following terms after completing the reading assignment. You should be able to cover the definition on the right and define the term out loud.

Annulus . . . . outer fibrous rim encircling the eardrum

Atresia . . . . congenital absence or closure of ear canal

Cerumen . . . . yellow, waxy material that lubricates and protects the ear canal

Cochlea . . . . inner ear structure containing the central hearing apparatus

Eustachian tube . . . . connects the middle ear with the nasopharynx and allows passage of air

Helix . . . . superior posterior free rim of the pinna

Incus . . . . "anvil," middle of the 3 ossicles of the middle ear

Malleus . . . . "hammer," first of the 3 ossicles of the middle ear

Mastoid . . . . bony prominence of the skull located just behind the ear

Organ of Corti . . . . sensory organ of hearing

Otalgia . . . . pain in the ear

Otitis externa . . . . inflammation of the outer ear and ear canal

Otitis media . . . . inflammation of the middle ear and tympanic membrane

Otorrhea . . . . discharge from the ear

Pars flaccida . . . . small, slack, superior section of tympanic membrane

Pars tensa . . . . thick, taut, central/inferior section of tympanic membrane

Pinna . . . . auricle, or outer ear

Stapes . . . . "stirrup," inner of the 3 ossicles of the middle ear

Tinnitus . . . . ringing in the ears

Tympanic membrane . . . . "eardrum," thin, translucent, oval membrane that stretches across the ear canal and separates the middle ear from the outer ear

Umbo . . . . knob of the malleus that shows through the tympanic membrane

Vertigo . . . . a spinning, twirling sensation

STUDY GUIDE

After completing the reading assignment and the media assignment, you should be able to answer the following questions in the spaces provided.

1. List the 3 functions of the middle ear.

2. Contrast 2 pathways of hearing.

3. Differentiate among the types of hearing loss, and give examples.

4. Relate the anatomic differences that place the infant at greater risk for middle ear infections.

5. Describe the whispered voice test of hearing acuity.

6. Explain the positioning of normal ear alignment in the child.

7. Define *otosclerosis* and *presbycusis*.

8. Contrast the motions used to straighten the ear canal when using the otoscope with an infant versus an adult.

9. Describe the appearance of these nodules that could be present on the external ear: Darwin's tubercle; sebaceous cyst; tophi; chondrodermatitis; keloid; carcinoma.

Jarvis, Carolyn: PHYSICAL EXAMINATION AND HEALTH ASSESSMENT: Sixth Edition,
Student Laboratory Manual. Copyright © 2012, 2008, 2004, 2000, 1996 by Saunders, an imprint of Elsevier Inc. All rights reserved.

10. Describe the appearance of these conditions that could appear in the ear canal: osteoma; exostosis; furuncle; polyp; foreign body.

11. List the disease state suggested by the following descriptions of the appearance of the eardrum: yellow-amber color; pearly gray color; air-fluid level; distorted light reflex; red color; dense white areas; oval dark areas; black or white dots on drum; blue drum.

12. List the findings that may appear during the whispered voice test and audiometric screening.

Fill in the labels indicated on the following illustrations.

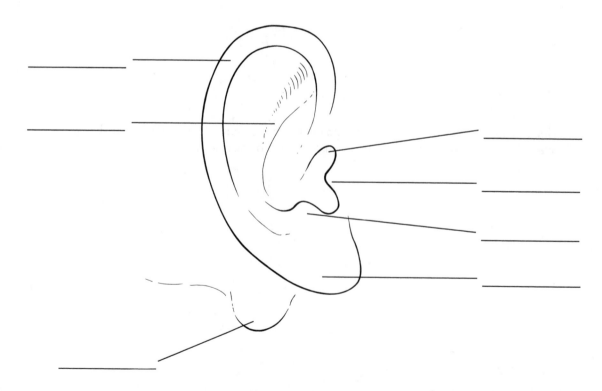

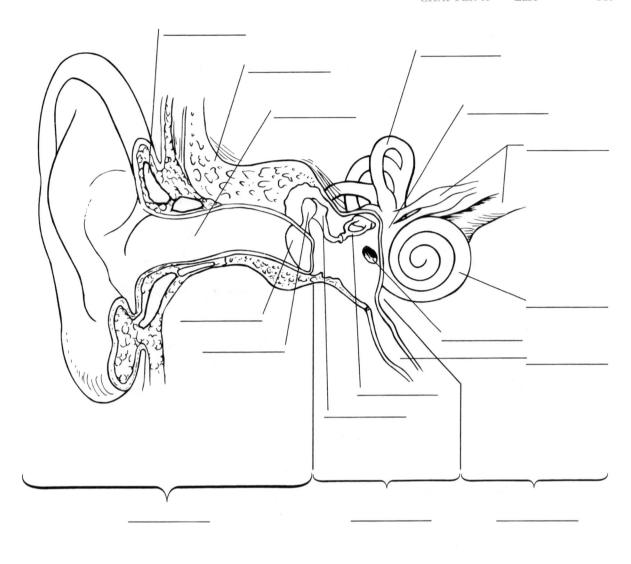

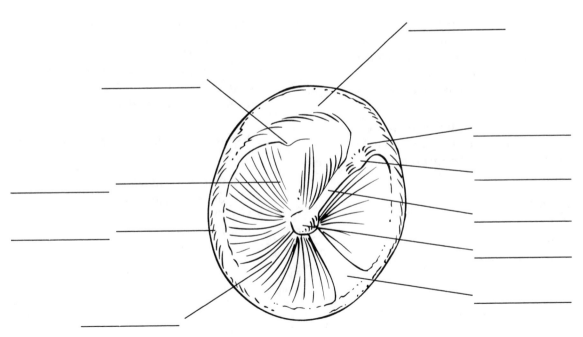

REVIEW QUESTIONS

This test is for you to check your own mastery of the content. Answers are provided in Appendix A.

1. Using the otoscope, the tympanic membrane is visualized. The color of a normal membrane is:

   a. deep pink.
   b. creamy white.
   c. pearly gray.
   d. dependent upon the ethnicity of the individual.

2. Sensorineural hearing loss may be related to:

   a. a gradual nerve degeneration.
   b. foreign bodies.
   c. impacted cerumen.
   d. perforated tympanic membrane.

3. Before examining the ear with the otoscope, the _____ should be palpated for tenderness.

   a. helix, external auditory meatus, and lobule
   b. mastoid process, tympanic membrane, and malleus
   c. pinna, pars flaccida, and antitragus
   d. pinna, tragus, and mastoid process

4. During the otoscopic examination of a child younger than 3 years, the examiner:

   a. pulls the pinna up and back.
   b. pulls the pinna down.
   c. holds the pinna gently but firmly in its normal position.
   d. tilts the head slightly toward the examiner.

5. While viewing with the otoscope, the examiner instructs the person to hold the nose and swallow. During this maneuver, the eardrum should:

   a. flutter.
   b. retract.
   c. bulge.
   d. remain immobile.

6. In examining the ear of an adult, the canal is straightened by pulling the auricle:

   a. down and forward.
   b. down and back.
   c. up and back.
   d. up and forward.

7. Darwin's tubercle is:

   a. an overgrowth of scar tissue.
   b. a blocked sebaceous gland.
   c. a sign of gout called *tophi*.
   d. a congenital, painless nodule at the helix.

8. When the ear is being examined with an otoscope, the patient's head should be:

   a. tilted toward the examiner.
   b. titled away from the examiner.
   c. as vertical as possible.
   d. tilted down.

9. The hearing receptors are located in the:

   a. vestibule.
   b. semicircular canals.
   c. middle ear.
   d. cochlea.

10. The sensation of vertigo is the result of:

    a. otitis media.
    b. pathology in the semicircular canals.
    c. pathology in the cochlea.
    d. 4th cranial nerve damage.

11. A common cause of a conductive hearing loss is:

    a. impacted cerumen.
    b. acute rheumatic fever.
    c. a CVA.
    d. otitis externa.

12. Upon examination of the tympanic membrane, visualization of which of the following findings indicates the infection of acute purulent otitis media?

   a. absent light reflex, bluish drum, oval dark areas
   b. absent light reflex, reddened drum, bulging drum
   c. oval dark areas on drum
   d. absent light reflex, air-fluid level, or bubbles behind drum
   e. retracted drum, very prominent landmarks

13. In examining a young adult woman, you observe her tympanic membrane to be yellow in color. You suspect she has:

   a. serum in the middle ear.
   b. blood in the middle ear.
   c. infection of the drumhead.
   d. jaundice.

14. Risk reduction for acute otitis media includes:

   a. use of pacifiers.
   b. increasing group daycare.
   c. avoiding breastfeeding.
   d. eliminating smoking in the house and car.

15. When assessing hearing acuity in a 6 month-old child, the examiner should:

   a. use an audiometer.
   b. observe for shyness and withdrawal.
   c. watch for head turning when saying the child's name.
   d. test the startle (Moro) reflex.

16. A patient with a head injury has clear, watery drainage from the ear; the examiner should:

   a. place a cotton ball loosely at the entrance to the ear canal.
   b. assess for the presence of glucose in the drainage.
   c. perform pneumatic otoscopy to assess for drum hypomobility.
   d. assess for the presence of a tympanostomy tube in the ear.

SKILLS LABORATORY/CLINICAL SETTING

You are now ready for the clinical component of the ear examination. The purpose of the clinical component is to practice the steps of the ear examination on a peer in the skills laboratory or on a patient in the clinical setting. The use of the otoscope is somewhat easier than the use of the ophthalmoscope; however, you still must be sure you are holding the instrument correctly. Holding the otoscope in an "upside down" position seems awkward at first, but it is important in order to make sure the otoscope tip does not cause pain to the delicate parts of the ear canal. Have someone correct your positioning before you insert the instrument.

Clinical Objectives

1. Collect a health history related to pertinent signs and symptoms of the ear system.

2. Describe the appearance of the normal outer ear and external ear canal.

3. Describe and demonstrate the correct technique of an otoscopic examination.

4. Describe and perform tests for hearing acuity.

5. Systematically describe the normal tympanic membrane including position, color, and landmarks.

6. Record the history and physical examination findings accurately, reach an assessment about the health state, and develop a plan of care.

Instructions

Prepare the examination setting and gather your equipment. Make certain the otoscope light is bright and batteries are freshly charged. Wash your hands. Practice the steps of the examination on a peer in the skills laboratory, giving appropriate instructions as you proceed. Record your findings using the regional write-up sheet that follows. The front of the page is intended as a worksheet; the back of the page is intended for your narrative summary recording using the SOAP format.

NOTES

REGIONAL WRITE-UP—EARS

Date _____

Examiner _____

Patient _____ Age _____ Gender _____

Reason for visit _____

I. Health History

	No	Yes, explain
1. Any **earache** or ear pain?		
2. Any ear **infections**?		
3. Any **discharge** from ears?		
4. Any **hearing loss**?		
5. Any **loud noises** at home or job?		
6. Any **ringing** or **buzzing** in ears?		
7. Ever felt **vertigo** (spinning)?		
8. How do you clean your ears?		

II. Physical Examination

A. Inspect and palpate external ear

Size and shape _____

Skin condition _____

Tenderness _____

External auditory meatus _____

B. Inspect using the otoscope

External canal _____

Tympanic membrane _____

Color and characteristics _____

Position _____

Integrity of membrane _____

C. Test hearing acuity

Whispered voice test _____

Pure tone audiometry _____

REGIONAL WRITE-UP—EARS

Summarize your findings using the SOAP format.

Subjective (Reason for seeking care, health history)

Objective (Physical examination findings)   Record findings on diagram below

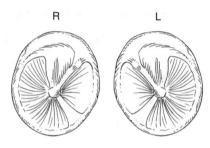

R   L

Assessment (Assessment of health state or problem, diagnosis)

Plan (Diagnostic evaluation, follow-up care, patient teaching)

Nose, Mouth, and Throat

PURPOSE

This chapter helps you learn the structure and function of the nose, mouth, and throat; learn the methods of inspection and palpation of these structures; and record the assessment accurately.

READING ASSIGNMENT

Jarvis: *Physical Examination and Health Assessment*, 6th ed., Chapter 16, pp. 351-382.

MEDIA ASSIGNMENT

Jarvis: *Physical Examination and Health Assessment* DVD Series: Nose, Mouth, Throat, and Neck.

GLOSSARY

Study the following terms after completing the reading assignment. You should be able to cover the definition on the right and define the term out loud.

Aphthous ulcers . . . . "canker sores"—small, painful, round ulcers in the oral mucosa of unknown cause

Buccal . . . . pertaining to the cheek

Candidiasis . . . . (moniliasis) white, cheesy, curdlike patch on buccal mucosa due to superficial fungal infection

Caries . . . . decay in the teeth

Cheilitis . . . . red, scaling, shallow, painful fissures at corners of mouth

Choanal atresia . . . . closure of nasal cavity due to congenital septum between nasal cavity and pharynx

Crypts . . . . indentations on surface of tonsils

Epistaxis . . . . nosebleed, usually from anterior septum

Epulis . . . . nontender, fibrous nodule of the gum

Fordyce granules . . . . small, isolated, white or yellow papules on oral mucosa

Gingivitis . . . . red, swollen gum margins that bleed easily

Herpes simplex . . . . "cold sores"—clear vesicles with red base that evolve into pustules, usually at lip-skin junction

Koplik spots . . . . small, blue-white spots with red halo over oral mucosa; early sign of measles

Leukoplakia . . . . chalky white, thick, raised patch on sides of tongue; precancerous

Malocclusion . . . . upper or lower dental arches out of alignment

Papillae . . . . rough, bumpy elevations on dorsal surface of tongue

Parotid glands . . . . pair of salivary glands in the cheeks in front of the ears

Pharyngitis . . . . inflammation of the throat

Plaque . . . . soft, whitish debris on teeth

Polyp . . . . smooth, pale gray nodules in the nasal cavity due to chronic allergic rhinitis

Rhinitis . . . . red, swollen inflammation of nasal mucosa

Thrush . . . . oral candidiasis in the newborn

Turbinate . . . . one of 3 bony projections into nasal cavity

Uvula . . . . free projection hanging down from the middle of the soft palate

STUDY GUIDE

After completing the reading assignment and the media assignment, you should be able to answer the following questions in the spaces provided.

1. Name the functions of the nose.

2. Describe the size and components of the nasal cavity.

3. List the 4 sets of paranasal sinuses, and describe their function.

4. List the 3 pairs of salivary glands, including their location and the locations of their duct openings.

5. After tooth loss in the middle or older adult, describe the consequences of chewing with the remaining maloccluded teeth.

6. Describe the appearance of a deviated nasal septum and a perforated septum.

7. Describe the appearance of a torus palatinus, and explain its significance.

8. Contrast the physical appearance and clinical significance of the following: leukoedema; candidiasis; leukoplakia; Fordyce granules.

Jarvis, Carolyn: PHYSICAL EXAMINATION AND HEALTH ASSESSMENT: Sixth Edition,
Student Laboratory Manual. Copyright © 2012, 2008, 2004, 2000, 1996 by Saunders, an imprint of Elsevier Inc. All rights reserved.

9. List the 4-point grading scale for the size of tonsils.

10. Describe the appearance and clinical significance of these findings in the infant: sucking tubercle; Epstein pearls; Bednar aphthae.

11. Contrast the appearance of nasal turbinates versus nasal polyps.

12. Describe the appearance and clinical significance of these findings on the tongue: ankyloglossia; fissured tongue; geographic tongue; black hairy tongue; macroglossia.

13. In the space below, sketch a cleft palate and a bifid uvula.

Fill in the labels indicated on the following illustrations.

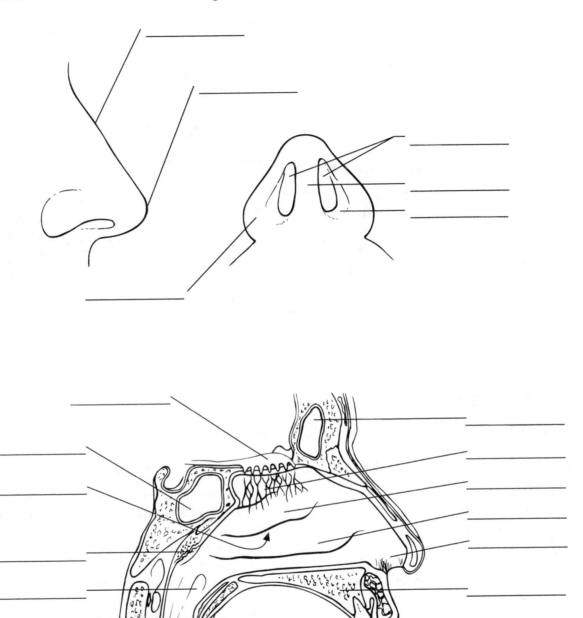

LEFT LATERAL WALL–NASAL CAVITY

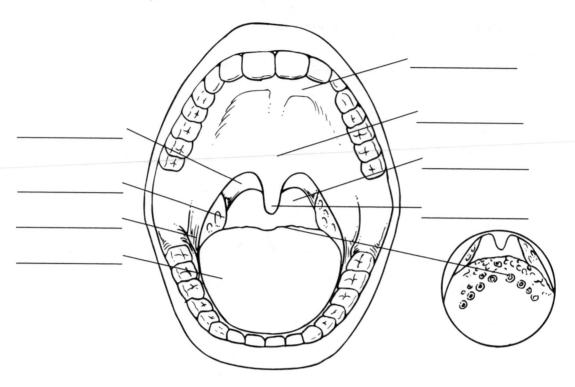

REVIEW QUESTIONS

This test is for you to check your own mastery of the content. Answers are provided in Appendix A.

1. The most common site of nosebleeds is:

   a. the turbinates.
   b. the columellae.
   c. Kiesselbach plexus.
   d. the meatus.

2. The sinuses that are accessible to examination are the:

   a. ethmoid and sphenoid.
   b. frontal and ethmoid.
   c. maxillary and sphenoid.
   d. frontal and maxillary.

3. The frenulum is:

   a. the midline fold of tissue that connects the tongue to the floor of the mouth.
   b. the anterior border of the oral cavity.
   c. the arching roof of the mouth.
   d. the free projection hanging down from the middle of the soft palate.

4. The largest salivary gland is located:

   a. within the cheeks in front of the ear.
   b. beneath the mandible at the angle of the jaw.
   c. within the floor of the mouth under the tongue.
   d. at the base of the tongue.

5. A 70-year-old woman complains of dry mouth. The most frequent cause of this problem is:

   a. the aging process.
   b. related to medications she may be taking.
   c. the use of dentures.
   d. related to a diminished sense of smell.

6. During an inspection of the nares, a deviated septum is noted. The best action is to:

   a. request a consultation with an ear, nose, and throat specialist.
   b. document the deviation in the medical record in case the person needs to be suctioned.
   c. teach the person what to do if a nosebleed should occur.
   d. explore further because polyps frequently accompany a deviated septum.

7. Oral malignancies are most likely to develop:

   a. on the soft palate.
   b. on the tongue.
   c. in the buccal cheek mucosa.
   d. in the mucosal "gutter" under the tongue.

8. In a medical record, the tonsils are graded as 3+. The tonsils would be:

   a. visible.
   b. halfway between the tonsillar pillars and uvula.
   c. touching the uvula.
   d. touching each other.

9. The function of the nasal turbinates is to:

   a. warm the inhaled air.
   b. detect odors.
   c. stimulate tear formation.
   d. lighten the weight of the skull bones.

10. The opening of an adult's parotid gland (Stensen's duct) is opposite the:

    a. lower 2nd molar.
    b. lower incisors.
    c. upper incisors.
    d. upper 2nd molar.

11. A nasal polyp may be distinguished from the nasal turbinates for 3 of the following reasons. Which reason is *false*?

    a. The polyp is highly vascular.
    b. The polyp is movable.
    c. The polyp is pale gray in color.
    d. The polyp is nontender.

12. The examiner notes small, round, white, shiny papules on the hard palate and gums of a 2-month-old. What is the significance of this finding?

    a. These are aphthous areas or ulcers that are the result of sucking.
    b. Teeth buds are beginning to appear.
    c. This is a normal finding called *Epstein pearls*.
    d. It indicates the presence of a monilial infection.

13. When assessing the tongue, the examiner should:

    a. palpate the U-shaped area under the tongue.
    b. check tongue color for cyanosis.
    c. use a tongue blade to elevate the tongue while placing your finger under the jaw.
    d. ask the person to say "ahhh" and note a rise in the midline.

SKILLS LABORATORY/CLINICAL SETTING

You are now ready for the clinical component of the nose, mouth, and throat examination. The purpose of the clinical component is to practice the steps of the examination on a peer in the skills laboratory or on a patient in the clinical setting and to achieve the following.

Clinical Objectives

1. Inspect the external nose.

2. Demonstrate use of the otoscope and nasal attachment to inspect the structures of the nasal cavity.

3. Demonstrate knowledge of infection control practices during inspection and palpation of structures of the mouth and pharynx.

4. Record the history and physical examination findings accurately, reach an assessment of the health state, and develop a plan of care.

Instructions

Prepare the examination setting, and gather your equipment. Wash your hands. Practice the steps of the examination on a peer in the skills laboratory, giving appropriate instructions as you proceed. Record your findings using the regional write-up sheet that follows. The front of the page is intended as a worksheet; the back of the page is intended for your narrative summary recording using the SOAP format.

NOTES

Jarvis, Carolyn: PHYSICAL EXAMINATION AND HEALTH ASSESSMENT: Sixth Edition,
Student Laboratory Manual. Copyright © 2012, 2008, 2004, 2000, 1996 by Saunders, an imprint of Elsevier Inc. All rights reserved.

REGIONAL WRITE-UP—NOSE, MOUTH, AND THROAT

Date _____

Examiner _____

Patient _____ Age _____ Gender _____

Reason for visit _____

I. Health History

A. Nose

	No	Yes, explain
1. Any nasal **discharge**?		
2. Unusually frequent or severe colds?		
3. Any **sinus pain** or sinusitis?		
4. Any **trauma** or injury to nose?		
5. Any **nosebleeds**? How often?		
6. Any **allergies** or hay fever?		
7. Any change in sense of smell?		

B. Mouth and throat

	No	Yes, explain
1. Any **sores** in mouth, tongue?		
2. Any **sore throat**? How often?		
3. Any **bleeding gums**?		
4. Any **toothache**?		
5. Any **hoarseness,** voice change?		
6. Any difficulty **swallowing**?		
7. Any change in sense of taste?		
8. Do you smoke? How much/day?		
9. Tell me about usual dental care.		

II. Physical Examination

A. Inspect and palpate the nose

Symmetry _____

Deformity, asymmetry, inflammation _____

Test patency of each nostril _____

Using a nasal speculum, note:

    Color of nasal mucosa _____

    Discharge, foreign body _____

    Septum: deviation, perforation, bleeding _____

    Turbinates: color, swelling, exudate, polyps _____

B. Palpate the sinus area

Frontal _____

Maxillary _____

C. Inspect the mouth

Lips _____

Teeth and gums _____

Buccal mucosa _____

Palate and uvula _____

Tonsils (grade) _____

Tongue _____

D. Inspect the throat

Tonsils: condition and grade _____

Pharyngeal wall _____

Any breath odor _____

REGIONAL WRITE-UP—NOSE, MOUTH, AND THROAT

Summarize your findings using the SOAP format.

Subjective (Reason for seeking care, health history)

Objective (Physical examination findings)

Record findings on diagram below

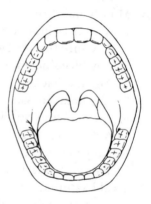

Assessment (Assessment of health state or problem, diagnosis)

Plan (Diagnostic evaluation, follow-up care, patient teaching)

Breasts and Regional Lymphatics

PURPOSE

This chapter helps you learn the structure and function of the breast; understand the rationale and methods of examination of the breast; accurately record the assessment; and teach breast self-examination.

READING ASSIGNMENT

Jarvis: *Physical Examination and Health Assessment*, 6th ed., Chapter 17, pp. 383-410.

MEDIA ASSIGNMENT

Jarvis: *Physical Examination and Health Assessment* DVD Series: Breasts and Regional Lymphatics.

GLOSSARY

Study the following terms after completing the reading assignment. You should be able to cover the definition on the right and define the term out loud.

Alveoli . . . . smallest structures of mammary gland

Areola . . . . darkened area surrounding nipple

Colostrum . . . . thin, yellow fluid, precursor of milk, secreted for a few days after birth

Cooper's ligaments . . . . suspensory ligaments; fibrous bands extending from the inner breast surface to the chest wall muscles

Fibroadenoma . . . . benign breast mass

Gynecomastia . . . . excessive breast development in the male

Intraductal papilloma . . . . serosanguineous nipple discharge

Inverted . . . . nipples that are depressed or invaginated

Lactiferous . . . . conveying milk

Mastalgia . . . . pain in breast

Mastitis . . . . inflammation of the breast

Montgomery's glands . . . . sebaceous glands in the areola, secrete protective lipid during lactation; also called *tubercles of Montgomery*

Paget's disease . . . . intraductal carcinoma in the breast

Peau d'orange. . . . . orange-peel appearance of breast due to edema

Retraction . . . . dimple or pucker on the skin

Striae . . . . atrophic pink, purple, or white linear streaks on the breasts, associated with pregnancy, excessive weight gain, or rapid growth during adolescence

Supernumerary nipple . . . . minute extra nipple along the embryonic milk line

Tail of Spence . . . . extension of breast tissue into the axilla

STUDY GUIDE

After completing the reading assignment and the media assignment, you should be able to answer the following questions in the spaces provided.

1. Identify appropriate history questions to ask regarding the breast examination.

2. Describe the anatomy of the breast.

3. Correlate changes in the female breast with normal developmental stages.

4. Describe the components of the breast examination.

5. List points to include in teaching the breast self-examination.

6. Explain the significance of a supernumerary nipple/breast.

7. Differentiate between the female and male examination procedure and findings.

8. Discuss pathologic changes that may occur in the breast:

   Benign breast disease _____

   Abscess _____

   Acute mastitis _____

   Fibroadenoma _____

   Cancer _____

   Paget's disease _____

9. List and describe the characteristics to consider when a mass is noted in the breast.

10. Define gynecomastia.

11. Describe screening mammography and clinical breast examination (CBE) for diagnosis of breast lesions.

12. List the high-risk and moderate-risk factors that increase the usual risk for breast cancer.

Fill in the labels on the following diagrams.

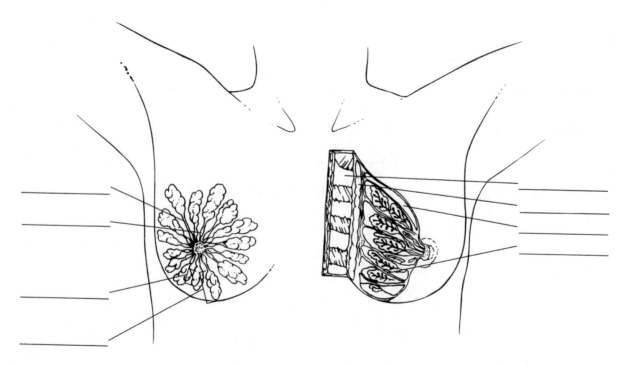

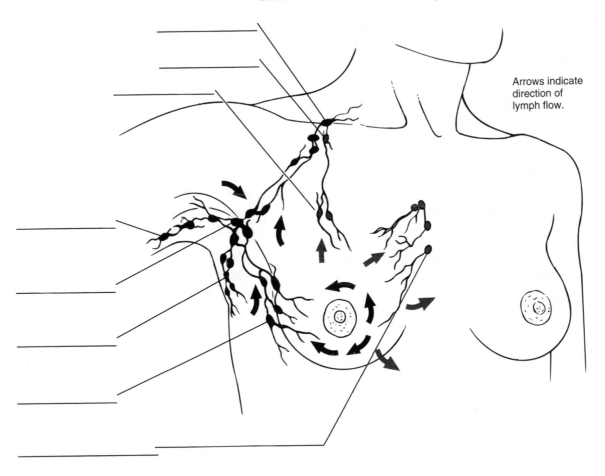

Arrows indicate direction of lymph flow.

REVIEW QUESTIONS

This test is for you to check your own mastery of the content. Answers are provided in Appendix A.

1. The reservoirs for storing milk in the breast are:

   a. lobules.
   b. alveoli.
   c. Montgomery's glands.
   d. lactiferous sinuses.

2. The most common site of breast tumors is:

   a. upper inner quadrant.
   b. upper outer quadrant.
   c. lower inner quadrant.
   d. lower outer quadrant.

3. During a visit for a school physical, the 13-year-old girl being examined questions the asymmetry of her breasts. The best response is:

   a. "One breast may grow faster than the other during development."
   b. "I will give you a referral for a mammogram."
   c. "You will probably have fibrocystic disease when you are older."
   d. "This may be an indication of hormonal imbalance. We will check again in 6 months."

4. When teaching the breast self-examination, you would inform the woman that the best time to conduct breast self-examination is:

   a. at the onset of the menstrual period.
   b. on the 14th day of the menstrual cycle.
   c. on the 4th to 7th day of the cycle.
   d. just before the menstrual period.

5. This is the first visit for a woman, age 38 years. The practitioner instructs her that a baseline mammogram is recommended for women between the ages of 35 and 39 years and that the clinical examination schedule would be based on age. The recommendation for women ages 40 to 49 years is:

   a. every year.
   b. every 2 years.
   c. twice a year.
   d. only the baseline examination is needed unless the woman has symptoms.

6. The examiner is going to inspect the breasts for retraction. The best position for this part of the examination is:

   a. lying supine with arms at the sides.
   b. leaning forward with hands outstretched.
   c. sitting with hand pushing onto hips.
   d. one arm at the side, the other arm elevated.

7. A bimanual technique may be the preferred approach for a woman:

   a. who is pregnant.
   b. who is having the first breast examination by a health care provider.
   c. with pendulous breasts.
   d. who has felt a change in the breast during self-examination.

8. During the examination of a 70-year-old man, you note gynecomastia. You would:

   a. refer for a biopsy.
   b. refer for a mammogram.
   c. review the medications for drugs that have gynecomastia as a side effect.
   d. proceed with the examination. This is a normal part of the aging process.

9. During a breast examination, you detect a mass. Identify the description that is most consistent with cancer rather than benign breast disease.

   a. round, firm, well demarcated
   b. irregular, poorly defined, fixed
   c. rubbery, mobile, tender
   d. lobular, clear margins, negative skin retraction

10. During the examination of the breasts of a pregnant woman, you would expect to find:

    a. peau d'orange.
    b. nipple retraction.
    c. a unilateral, obvious venous pattern.
    d. a blue vascular pattern over both breasts.

11. Which of the following women should not be referred to a physician for further evaluation?

    a. a 26-year-old with multiple nodules palpated in each breast
    b. a 48-year-old who has a 6-month history of reddened and sore left nipple and areolar area
    c. a 25-year-old with asymmetric breasts and inversion of nipples since adolescence
    d. a 64-year-old with ulcerated area at tip of right nipple; no masses, tenderness, or lymph nodes palpated

12. Breast asymmetry:

    a. increases with age and parity.
    b. may be normal.
    c. indicates a neoplasm.
    d. is accompanied by enlarged axillary lymph nodes.

13. Any lump found in the breast should be referred for further evaluation. A benign lesion will usually have 3 of the following characteristics. Which one is characteristic of a malignant lesion?

    a. soft
    b. well-defined margins
    c. freely movable
    d. irregular shape

14. Gynecomastia is:

    a. enlargement of the male breast.
    b. presence of "mast" cells in the male breast.
    c. cancer of the male breast.
    d. presence of supernumerary breast on the male chest.

15. Which is the first physical change associated with puberty in girls?

    a. areolar elevation
    b. breast bud development
    c. height spurt
    d. pubic hair development
    e. menarche

16. During the examination of a 30-year-old woman, she questions you about "the 2 large moles" that are below her left breast. After examining the area, how do you respond?

    a. "I think you should be examined by a dermatologist."
    b. "This appears to be a normal finding of supernumerary nipples, due to the small areolae and nipples that are present."
    c. "These are Montgomery's glands, which are common."
    d. "Is there a possibility you are pregnant?"

17. The breasts of a neonate may be large and very visible, secreting clear or white fluid. What is the basis of this finding?

    a. It may be due to birth trauma.
    b. The fluid is colostrum, which is typically seen as a precursor to milk.
    c. The cause is maternal estrogen, which crossed the placenta.
    d. This often occurs with premature thelarche.

SKILLS LABORATORY/CLINICAL SETTING

You are now ready for the clinical component of the breast assessment. The purpose of the clinical component is to practice the steps of the assessment on a peer in the skills laboratory and to achieve the following.

Clinical Objectives

1. Demonstrate knowledge of the symptoms related to the breasts and axillae by obtaining a health history.

2. Perform inspection and palpation of the breasts, with the woman in sitting and supine positions, using proper technique and providing appropriate draping.

3. Teach the breast self-examination to a woman, or list the points to include in teaching the breast self-examination.

4. Record the history and physical examination findings accurately, reach an assessment of the health state, and develop a plan of care.

Instructions

Practice the steps of the breast examination on a peer or on a woman in the clinical area. Record your findings on the regional write-up sheet that follows. The front of the page is intended as a worksheet; the back of the page is intended for your narrative summary recording using the SOAP format.

Note the student performance checklist that follows the regional write-up sheet. It lists the essential behaviors you should display as an examiner, and it may be used by your clinical instructor to evaluate your clinical teaching of breast self-examination.

NOTES

REGIONAL WRITE-UP—BREASTS AND AXILLAE

Date _____

Examiner _____

Patient _____ Age _____ Gender _____

Reason for visit _____

I. Health History

	No	Yes, explain
1. Any **pain** or tenderness in breasts?		
2. Any **lump** or thickening in breasts?		
3. Any **discharge** from nipples?		
4. Any **rash** on breasts?		
5. Any **swelling** in the breasts?		
6. Any **trauma** or injury to breasts?		
7. Any **history** of breast disease?		
8. Ever had **surgery** on breasts?		
9. Ever been taught breast self-examination?		
10. Ever had mammography?		

II. Physical Examination

A. Inspection

1. Breasts

   Symmetry _____

   Skin color and condition _____

   Texture _____

   Lesions _____

2. Areolae and nipples

   Shape _____

   Direction _____

   Surface characteristics _____

   Discharge _____

3. Response to arm movement _____

4. Axillae _____

B. Palpation

1. Breasts

   Texture _____

   Masses _____

   Tenderness _____

2. Areolae and nipples

   Masses _____

   Discharge _____

3. Axillae and lymph nodes

   Size _____

   Shape _____

   Consistency _____

   Mobility _____

   Discrete or matted _____

   Tenderness _____

C. Teach breast self-examination

REGIONAL WRITE-UP—BREASTS AND AXILLAE

Summarize your findings using the SOAP format.

Subjective (Reason for seeking care, health history)

Objective (Physical examination findings)

Record findings on diagram below

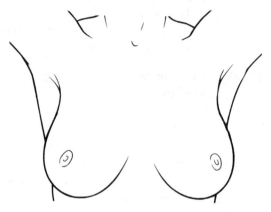

Assessment (Assessment of health state or problem, diagnosis)

Plan (Diagnostic evaluation, follow-up care, teaching)

STUDENT COMPETENCY CHECKLIST

TEACHING BREAST SELF-EXAMINATION (BSE)

	S	U	Comments
A. Cognitive			
1. Explain:			
a. why breasts are examined			
(1) in the shower			
(2) before a mirror			
(3) supine with pillow under side of breast being examined			
b. who should do breast examination			
c. frequency of breast examination			
d. best time of the month to do breast examination and rationale			
2. State the area of breast where most lumps are found			
3. Give two reasons a person may not report significant findings to the health care provider			
B. Performance			
1. Explains to woman need for BSE			
2. Instructs woman on technique of BSE by:			
a. inspecting and bilaterally comparing breasts in front of mirror			
b. noting new or unusual rash or redness on skin and areola			
c. palpating breast in a systemic manner, using pads of three fingers and with woman's arm raised overhead			
d. palpating tail of Spence and axilla			
e. gently compressing nipples			
3. Instructs woman to report unusual findings to the health professional at once			
4. Asks woman to do return demonstration			

NOTES

PURPOSE

This chapter helps you learn the structure and function of the thorax and lungs; understand the methods of examination of the respiratory system; identify lung sounds that are normal; describe the characteristics of adventitious lung sounds; and accurately record the assessment. At the end of this unit you will be able to perform a complete physical examination of the respiratory system.

READING ASSIGNMENT

Jarvis: *Physical Examination and Health Assessment*, 6th ed., Chapter 18, pp. 411-454.

MEDIA ASSIGNMENT

Jarvis: *Physical Examination and Health Assessment* DVD Series: Thorax and Lungs.

GLOSSARY

Study the following terms after completing the reading assignment. You should be able to cover the definition on the right and define the term out loud.

Alveoli . . . . functional units of the lung; the thin-walled chambers surrounded by networks of capillaries that are the site of respiratory exchange of carbon dioxide and oxygen

Angle of Louis . . . . manubriosternal angle, the articulation of the manubrium and body of the sternum, continuous with the second rib

Apnea . . . . cessation of breathing

Asthma . . . . an abnormal respiratory condition associated with allergic hypersensitivity to certain inhaled allergens, characterized by bronchospasm, wheezing, and dyspnea

Atelectasis . . . . an abnormal respiratory condition characterized by collapsed, shrunken, deflated section of alveoli

Bradypnea . . . . slow breathing, <10 breaths per minute, regular rate

Bronchiole...................one of the smaller respiratory passageways into which the segmental bronchi divide

Bronchitis.................inflammation of the bronchi with partial obstruction of bronchi due to excessive mucus secretion

Bronchophony..............the spoken voice sound heard through the stethoscope, which sounds soft, muffled, and indistinct over normal lung tissue

Bronchovesicular...........the normal breath sound heard over major bronchi, characterized by moderate pitch and an equal duration of inspiration and expiration

Chronic obstructive pulmonary disease (COPD)...a functional category of abnormal respiratory conditions characterized by airflow obstruction (e.g., emphysema, chronic bronchitis)

Cilia.....................millions of hairlike cells lining the tracheobronchial tree

Consolidation..............the solidification of portions of lung tissue as it fills up with infectious exudate, as in pneumonia

Crackles...................(rales) abnormal, discontinuous, adventitious lung sounds heard on inspiration

Crepitus...................coarse, crackling sensation palpable over the skin when air abnormally escapes from the lung and enters the subcutaneous tissue

Dead space.................passageways that transport air but are not available for gaseous exchange (e.g., trachea, bronchi)

Dyspnea...................difficult, labored breathing

Egophony..................the voice sound of "eeeeee" heard through the stethoscope

Emphysema................the chronic obstructive pulmonary disease characterized by enlargement of alveoli distal to terminal bronchioles

Fissure...................the narrow crack dividing the lobes of the lungs

Fremitus...................a palpable vibration from the spoken voice felt over the chest wall

Friction rub...............a coarse, grating, adventitious lung sound heard when the pleurae are inflamed

Hypercapnia..............(hypercarbia) increased levels of carbon dioxide in the blood

Hyperventilation...........increased rate and depth of breathing

Hypoxemia................decreased level of oxygen in the blood

Intercostal space...........space between the ribs

Kussmaul respiration.......a type of hyperventilation that occurs with diabetic ketoacidosis

Orthopnea.................ability to breathe easily only in an upright position

Paroxysmal nocturnal dyspnea...................sudden awakening from sleeping with shortness of breath

Percussion................striking over the chest wall with short, sharp blows of the fingers to determine the size and density of the underlying organ

Pleural effusion...........abnormal fluid between the layers of the pleura

Rhonchi...................low-pitched, musical, snoring, adventitious lung sound caused by airflow obstruction from secretions

Jarvis, Carolyn: PHYSICAL EXAMINATION AND HEALTH ASSESSMENT: Sixth Edition, Student Laboratory Manual. Copyright © 2012, 2008, 2004, 2000, 1996 by Saunders, an imprint of Elsevier Inc. All rights reserved.

Tachypnea . . . . rapid, shallow breathing, >24 breaths per minute

Vesicular . . . . the soft, low-pitched, normal breath sounds heard over peripheral lung fields

Vital capacity . . . . the amount of air following maximal inspiration that can be exhaled

Wheeze . . . . high-pitched, musical, squeaking adventitious lung sound

Whispered pectoriloquy . . . . . . a whispered phrase heard through the stethoscope that sounds faint and inaudible over normal lung tissue

Xiphoid process . . . . sword-shaped lower tip of the sternum

STUDY GUIDE

After completing the reading assignment and the media assignment, you should be able to answer the following questions in the spaces provided.

1. Describe the most important points about the health history for the respiratory system.

2. Describe the pleura and its function.

3. List the structures that compose the respiratory dead space.

4. Summarize the mechanics of respiration.

Jarvis, Carolyn: PHYSICAL EXAMINATION AND HEALTH ASSESSMENT: Sixth Edition,
Student Laboratory Manual. Copyright © 2012, 2008, 2004, 2000, 1996 by Saunders, an imprint of Elsevier Inc. All rights reserved.

5. List the elements included in the inspection of the respiratory system.

6. Discuss the significance of a "barrel chest."

7. List and describe common thoracic deformities.

8. List and describe 3 types of normal breath sounds.

9. Define 2 types of adventitious breath sounds.

10. The manubriosternal angle is also called _____.

    Why is it a useful landmark?

11. How many degrees is the normal costal angle? _____

12. When comparing the anteroposterior diameter of the chest with the transverse diameter, what is the expected ratio?

    What is the significance of this?

13. What is tripod position?

14. List 3 factors that affect normal intensity of tactile fremitus.

    1. _____

    2. _____

    3. _____

15. During percussion, which sound would you expect to predominate over normal lung tissue?

16. Normal findings for diaphragmatic excursion are:

17. List 5 factors that can cause extraneous noise during auscultation.

    1. _____

    2. _____

    3. _____

    4. _____

    5. _____

18. Describe the 3 types of normal breath sounds.

Name   Location   Description

_____

_____

_____

Fill in the labels indicated on the following illustration.

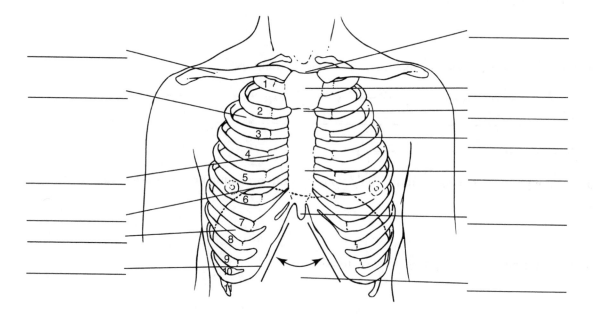

Draw in the lobes of the lungs and label their landmarks on the following two illustrations.

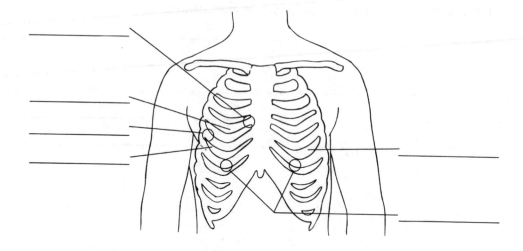

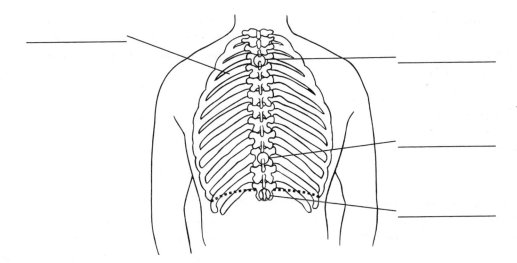

REVIEW QUESTIONS

This test is for you to check your own mastery of the content. Answers are provided in Appendix A.

1. The manubriosternal angle is:

   a. the articulation of the manubrium and the body of the sternum.
   b. a hollow, U-shaped depression just above the sternum.
   c. also known as the *breastbone.*
   d. a term synonymous with costochondral junction.

2. Select the correct description of the left lung.

   a. narrower than the right lung with three lobes
   b. narrower than the right lung with two lobes
   c. wider than the right lung with two lobes
   d. shorter than the right lung with three lobes

3. Some conditions have a cough with characteristic timing. The cough associated with chronic bronchitis is best described as:

   a. continuous throughout the day.
   b. productive cough for at least 3 months of the year for 2 years in a row.
   c. occurring in the afternoon/evening because of exposure to irritants at work.
   d. occurring in the early morning.

4. Symmetric chest expansion is best confirmed by:

   a. placing hands on the posterolateral chest wall with thumbs at the level of T9 or T10 and then sliding the hands up to pinch up a small fold of skin between the thumbs.
   b. inspection of the shape and configuration of the chest wall.
   c. placing the palmar surface of the fingers of one hand against the chest and having the person repeat the words "ninety-nine."
   d. percussion of the posterior chest.

5. Absence of diaphragmatic excursion occurs with:

   a. asthma.
   b. an unusually thick chest wall.
   c. pleural effusion or atelectasis of the lower lobes.
   d. age-related changes in the chest wall.

6. Auscultation of breath sounds is an important component of respiratory assessment. Select the most accurate description of this part of the examination.

   a. Hold the bell of the stethoscope against the chest wall; listen to the entire right field and then the entire left field.
   b. Hold the diaphragm of the stethoscope against the chest wall; listen to one full respiration in each location, being sure to do side-to-side comparisons.
   c. Listen from the apices to the bases of each lung field using the bell of the stethoscope.
   d. Select the bell or diaphragm depending upon the quality of sounds heard; listen for one respiration in each location, moving from side to side.

7. Select the best description of bronchovesicular breath sounds:

   a. high pitched, of longer duration on inspiration than expiration.
   b. moderate pitched, inspiration equal to expiration.
   c. low pitched, inspiration greater than expiration.
   d. rustling sound, like the wind in the trees.

8. After examining a patient, you make the following notation: Increased respiratory rate, chest expansion decreased on left side, dull to percussion over left lower lobe, breath sounds louder with fine crackles over left lower lobe. These findings are consistent with a diagnosis of:

   a. bronchitis.
   b. asthma.
   c. pleural effusion.
   d. lobar pneumonia.

9. Upon examining a patient's nails, you note that the angle of the nail base is >160 degrees and that the nail base feels spongy to palpation. These findings are consistent with:

   a. adult respiratory distress syndrome.
   b. normal findings for the nails.
   c. chronic congenital heart disease and COPD.
   d. atelectasis.

10. Upon examination of a patient, you note a coarse, low-pitched sound during both inspiration and expiration. This patient complains of pain with breathing. These findings are consistent with:

    a. fine crackles.
    b. wheezes.
    c. atelectatic crackles.
    d. pleural friction rub.

11. In order to use the technique of egophony, ask the patient to:

    a. take several deep breaths and then hold for 5 seconds.
    b. say "eeeeee" each time the stethoscope is moved.
    c. repeat the phrase "ninety-nine" each time the stethoscope is moved.
    d. whisper a phrase as auscultation is performed.

12. When examining for tactile fremitus, it is important to:

    a. have the patient breathe quickly.
    b. ask the patient to cough.
    c. palpate the chest symmetrically.
    d. use the bell of the stethoscope.

13. The pulse oximeter measures:

    a. arterial oxygen saturation.
    b. venous oxygen saturation.
    c. combined saturation of arterial and venous blood.
    d. carboxyhemoglobin levels.

14. A pleural friction rub is best detected by:

    a. observation.
    b. palpation.
    c. auscultation.
    d. percussion.

15. A barrel-shaped chest is characterized by:

    a. equal anteroposterior-to-transverse diameter and ribs being horizontal.
    b. anteroposterior-to-transverse diameter of 1:2 and an elliptical shape.
    c. anteroposterior-to-transverse diameter of 2:1 and ribs being elevated.
    d. anteroposterior-to-transverse diameter of 3:7 and ribs sloping back.

Match column A to column B.

Column A—Lung borders

16. _____ apex

17. _____ base

18. _____ lateral left

19. _____ lateral right

20. _____ posterior apex

Column B—Location

a. rests on the diaphragm

b. C7

c. sixth rib, midclavicular line

d. fifth intercostal

e. 3 to 4 cm above the inner third of the clavicles

Match column A to column B.

Column A—Configurations of the thorax

21. _____ normal chest

22. _____ barrel chest

23. _____ pectus excavatum

24. _____ pectus carinatum

25. _____ scoliosis

26. _____ kyphosis

Column B—Description

a. anteroposterior = transverse diameter

b. exaggerated posterior curvature of thoracic spine

c. lateral S-shaped curvature of the thoracic and lumbar spine

d. sunken sternum and adjacent cartilages

e. elliptical shape with an anteroposterior:transverse diameter in the ratio of 1:2

f. forward protrusion of the sternum with ribs sloping back at either side

SKILLS LABORATORY/CLINICAL SETTING

You are now ready for the clinical component of the respiratory system. The purpose of the clinical component is to practice the regional examination on a peer in the skills laboratory or on a patient in the clinical setting and to achieve the following.

Clinical Objectives

1. Demonstrate knowledge of the symptoms related to the respiratory system by obtaining a regional health history from a peer/patient.

2. Correctly locate anatomic landmarks on the thorax of a peer.

3. Using a grease pencil and with peer's permission, draw lobes of the lungs on a peer's thorax.

4. Demonstrate correct techniques for inspection, palpation, percussion, and auscultation of the respiratory system.

5. Demonstrate the technique for estimation of diaphragmatic excursion.

6. Record the history and physical examination findings accurately, reach an assessment of the health state, and develop a plan of care.

Instructions

Gather your equipment. Wash your hands. Clean the stethoscope endpiece with an alcohol wipe. Practice the steps of the examination of the thorax and lungs on a peer or on a patient in the clinical area. Record your findings using the regional write-up sheet. The front of the sheet is intended as a worksheet; the back of the sheet is intended for a narrative summary using the SOAP format.

NOTES

REGIONAL WRITE-UP—THORAX AND LUNGS

Date _____

Examiner _____

Patient _____ Age _____ Gender _____

Reason for visit _____

I. Health History

	No	Yes, explain
1. Do you have a **cough?**		
2. Any shortness of **breath?**		
3. Any **chest pain** with breathing?		
4. Any **past history** of lung diseases?		
5. Ever **smoke** cigarettes? How many/day? For how long?		
6. Any living or work conditions that affect your breathing?		
7. Last TB skin test, chest x-ray, flu vaccine?		

II. Physical Examination

A. Inspection

1. Thoracic cage _____

2. Respiratory rate and pattern _____

3. Skin _____

4. Person's position _____

5. Person's facial expression _____

6. Level of consciousness _____

B. Palpation

1. Confirm symmetric chest expansion _____

2. Tactile fremitus _____

3. Detect any lumps, masses, tenderness _____

4. Trachea _____

C. Percussion

1. Determine percussion note that predominates over lung fields _____

2. Diaphragmatic excursion _____

D. Auscultation

1. Listen: posterior, lateral, anterior _____

2. Any abnormal breath sounds? _____

   If so, perform bronchophony, _____

   whispered pectoriloquy, _____

   egophony _____

3. Any adventitious sounds? _____

REGIONAL WRITE-UP—THORAX AND LUNGS

Summarize your findings using the SOAP format.

Subjective (Reason for seeking care, health history)

Objective (Physical examination findings)   Use the drawing to record your findings

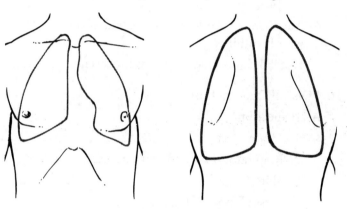

Assessment (Assessment of health state or problem, diagnosis)

Plan (Diagnostic evaluation, follow-up care, teaching)

PURPOSE

This chapter helps you learn the structure and function of the heart, valves, and great vessels; understand the cardiac cycle; describe the heart sounds; understand the rationale and methods of examination of the heart; and accurately record the assessment. At the end of this chapter you should be able to perform a complete assessment of the heart and neck vessels.

READING ASSIGNMENT

Jarvis: *Physical Examination and Health Assessment*, 6th ed., Chapter 19, pp. 455-498.

MEDIA ASSIGNMENT

Jarvis: *Physical Examination and Health Assessment* DVD Series: Cardiovascular System: Heart and Neck Vessels.

Google the Internet with the term *heart sounds*. Listen to several websites for a good sampling of the most common heart sounds you will encounter.

GLOSSARY

Study the following terms after completing the reading assignment. You should be able to cover the definition on the right and define the term out loud.

Angina pectoris . . . . acute chest pain that occurs when myocardial demand exceeds its oxygen supply

Aortic regurgitation . . . . (aortic insufficiency) incompetent aortic valve that allows backward flow of blood into left ventricle during diastole

Aortic stenosis . . . . calcification of aortic valve cusps that restricts forward flow of blood during systole

Aortic valve . . . . the left semilunar valve separating the left ventricle and the aorta

Apex of the heart . . . . tip of the heart pointing down toward the 5th left intercostal space

Apical impulse . . . . (point of maximal impulse, PMI) pulsation created as the left ventricle rotates against the chest wall during systole, normally at the 5th left intercostal space in the midclavicular line

Base of the heart . . . . broader area of heart's outline located at the 3rd right and left intercostal space

Bell (of the stethoscope) . . . . . . cup-shaped endpiece used for soft, low-pitched heart sounds

Bradycardia . . . . slow heart rate, <50 beats per minute in the adult

Clubbing . . . . bulbous enlargement of distal phalanges of fingers and toes that occurs with chronic cyanotic heart and lung conditions

Coarctation of aorta . . . . severe narrowing of the descending aorta, a congenital heart defect

Cor pulmonale . . . . right ventricular hypertrophy and heart failure due to pulmonary hypertension

Cyanosis . . . . dusky blue mottling of the skin and mucous membranes due to excessive amount of reduced hemoglobin in the blood

Diaphragm (of the stethoscope) . . . . flat endpiece of the stethoscope used for hearing relatively high-pitched heart sounds

Diastole . . . . the heart's filling phase

Dyspnea . . . . difficult, labored breathing

Edema . . . . swelling of legs or dependent body part due to increased interstitial fluid

Erb's point . . . . traditional auscultatory area in the 3rd left intercostal space

First heart sound (S_1) . . . . occurs with closure of the atrioventricular (AV) valves signaling the beginning of systole

Fourth heart sound (S_4) . . . . . . (S_4 gallop; atrial gallop) very soft, low-pitched ventricular filling sound that occurs in late diastole

Gallop rhythm . . . . the addition of a 3rd or a 4th heart sound makes the rhythm sound like the cadence of a galloping horse

Inching . . . . technique of moving the stethoscope incrementally across the precordium through the auscultatory areas while listening to the heart sounds

LVH (left ventricular hypertrophy) . . . . increase in thickness of myocardial wall that occurs when the heart pumps against chronic outflow obstruction (e.g., aortic stenosis)

MCL (midclavicular line) . . . . . imaginary vertical line bisecting the middle of the clavicle in each hemithorax

Mitral regurgitation . . . . (mitral insufficiency) incompetent mitral valve allows regurgitation of blood back into left atrium during systole

Mitral stenosis . . . . calcified mitral valve impedes forward flow of blood into left ventricle during diastole

Mitral valve . . . . left AV valve separating the left atria and ventricle

Palpitation . . . . uncomfortable awareness of rapid or irregular heart rate

Paradoxical splitting . . . . opposite of a normal split S$_2$ so that the split is heard in expiration, and in inspiration the sounds fuse to one sound

Pericardial friction rub . . . . high-pitched, scratchy extracardiac sound heard when the precordium is inflamed

Physiologic splitting . . . . normal variation in S$_2$ heard as two separate components during inspiration

Precordium . . . . area of the chest wall overlying the heart and great vessels

Pulmonic regurgitation . . . . (pulmonic insufficiency) backflow of blood through incompetent pulmonic valve into the right ventricle

Pulmonic stenosis . . . . calcification of pulmonic valve that restricts forward flow of blood during systole

Pulmonic valve . . . . right semilunar valve separating the right ventricle and pulmonary artery

Second heart sound (S$_2$) . . . . . . occurs with closure of the semilunar valves, aortic and pulmonic, and signals the end of systole

Summation gallop . . . . abnormal mid-diastolic heart sound heard when both the pathologic S$_3$ and S$_4$ are present

Syncope . . . . temporary loss of consciousness due to decreased cerebral blood flow (fainting), caused by ventricular asystole, pronounced bradycardia, or ventricular fibrillation

Systole . . . . the heart's pumping phase

Tachycardia . . . . rapid heart rate, >90 beats per minute in the adult

Third heart sound (S$_3$) . . . . soft, low-pitched ventricular filling sound that occurs in early diastole (S$_3$ gallop) and may be an early sign of heart failure

Thrill . . . . palpable vibration on the chest wall accompanying severe heart murmur

Tricuspid valve . . . . right AV valve separating the right atria and ventricle

STUDY GUIDE

After completing the reading assignment and the media assignment, you should be able to answer the following questions in the spaces provided.

1. Define the apical impulse and describe its normal location, size, and duration.

Which *normal* variations may affect the location of the apical impulse?

Which *abnormal* conditions may affect the location of the apical impulse?

2. Explain the mechanism producing normal first and second heart sounds.

3. Describe the effect of respiration on the heart sounds.

4. Describe the characteristics of the **first heart sound** and its intensity at the apex of the heart and at the base.

Which conditions *increase* the intensity of S_1?

Which conditions *decrease* the intensity of S_1?

5. Describe the characteristics of the **second heart sound** and its intensity at the apex of the heart and at the base.

Which conditions *increase* the intensity of S_2?

Which conditions *decrease* the intensity of S_2?

6. Explain the physiologic mechanism for normal splitting of S_2 in the pulmonic valve area.

7. Define the **third heart sound.** When in the cardiac cycle does it occur? Describe its intensity, quality, location in which it is heard, and method of auscultation.

8. Differentiate a physiologic S_3 from a pathologic S_3.

9. Define the **fourth heart sound.** When in the cardiac cycle does it occur? Describe its intensity, quality, location in which it is heard, and method of auscultation.

10. Explain the position of the valves during each phase of the cardiac cycle.

11. Define venous pressure and jugular venous pulse.

12. Differentiate between the carotid artery pulsation and the jugular vein pulsation.

—

13. List the areas of questioning to address during the health history of the cardiovascular system.

14. Define bruit, and discuss what it indicates.

15. Define heave or lift, and discuss what it indicates.

16. State 4 guidelines to distinguish S_1 from S_2.

    1. _____

    2. _____

    3. _____

    4. _____

17. Define pulse deficit, and discuss what it indicates.

18. Define preload and afterload.

19. List the characteristics to explore when you hear a murmur, including the grading scale of murmurs.

20. Discuss the characteristics of an innocent or functional murmur.

Fill in the labels indicated on the following illustrations.

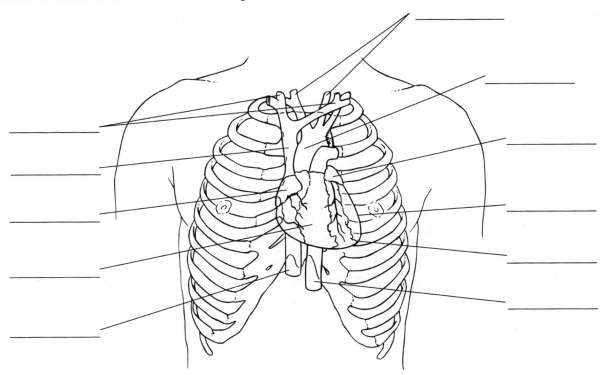

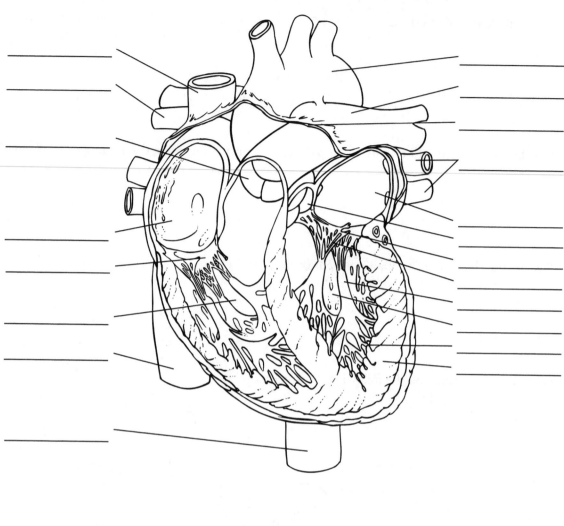

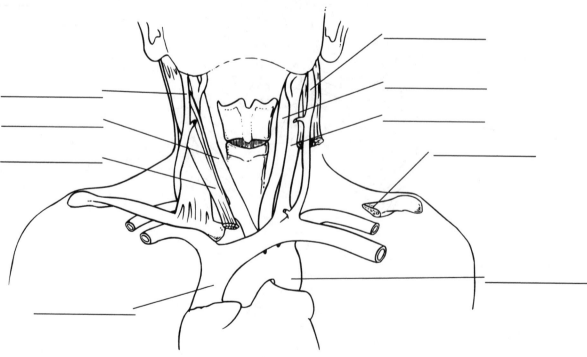

REVIEW QUESTIONS

This test is for you to check your own mastery of the content. Answers are provided in Appendix A.

1. The precordium is:

   a. a synonym for the mediastinum.
   b. the area on the chest where the apical impulse is felt.
   c. the area on the anterior chest overlying the heart and great vessels.
   d. a synonym for the area where the superior and inferior venae cavae return unoxygenated venous blood to the right side of the heart.

2. Select the best description of the tricuspid valve.

   a. left semilunar valve
   b. right atrioventricular valve
   c. left atrioventricular valve
   d. right semilunar valve

3. The function of the pulmonic valve is to:

   a. divide the left atrium and left ventricle.
   b. guard the opening between the right atrium and right ventricle.
   c. protect the orifice between the right ventricle and the pulmonary artery.
   d. guard the entrance to the aorta from the left ventricle.

4. Atrial systole occurs:

   a. during ventricular systole.
   b. during ventricular diastole.
   c. concurrently with ventricular systole.
   d. independently of ventricular function.

5. The second heart sound is the result of:

   a. opening of the mitral and tricuspid valves.
   b. closing of the mitral and tricuspid valves.
   c. opening of the aortic and pulmonic valves.
   d. closing of the aortic and pulmonic valves.

6. The examiner has estimated the jugular venous pressure. Identify the finding that is abnormal.

   a. patient elevated to 30 degrees, internal jugular vein pulsation at 1 cm above sternal angle
   b. patient elevated to 30 degrees, internal jugular vein pulsation at 2 cm above sternal angle
   c. patient elevated to 40 degrees, internal jugular vein pulsation at 1 cm above sternal angle
   d. patient elevated to 45 degrees, internal jugular vein pulsation at 4 cm above sternal angle

7. The examiner is palpating the apical impulse. The normal size of this impulse:

   a. is less than 1 cm.
   b. is about 2 cm.
   c. is 3 cm.
   d. varies depending on the size of the person.

8. The examiner wishes to listen in the pulmonic valve area. To do this, the stethoscope would be placed at the:

   a. second right interspace.
   b. second left interspace.
   c. left lower sternal border.
   d. fifth interspace, left midclavicular line.

9. Select the statement that best differentiates a split S_2 from S_3.

   a. S_3 is lower pitched and is heard at the apex.
   b. S_2 is heard at the left lower sternal border.
   c. The timing of S_2 varies with respirations.
   d. S_3 is heard at the base; timing varies with respirations.

10. The examiner wishes to listen for a pericardial friction rub. Select the best method of listening.

    a. with the diaphragm, patient sitting up and leaning forward, breath held in expiration
    b. using the bell with the patient leaning forward
    c. at the base during normal respiration
    d. with the diaphragm, patient turned to the left side

11. When auscultating the heart, your first step is to:

    a. identify S_1 and S_2.
    b. listen for S_3 and S_4.
    c. listen for murmurs.
    d. identify all four sounds on the first round.

12. You will hear a split S_2 most clearly in what area?

    a. apical
    b. pulmonic
    c. tricuspid
    d. aortic

13. The stethoscope bell should be pressed lightly against the skin so that:

    a. chest hair doesn't simulate crackles.
    b. high-pitched sounds can be heard better.
    c. it does not act as a diaphragm.
    d. it does not interfere with amplification of heart sounds.

14. A murmur heard after S_1 and before S_2 is classified as:

    a. diastolic (possibly benign).
    b. diastolic (always pathologic).
    c. systolic (possibly benign).
    d. systolic (always pathologic).

15. When assessing the carotid artery, the examiner should palpate:

    a. bilaterally at the same time, while standing behind the patient.
    b. medial to the sternomastoid muscle, one side at a time.
    c. for a bruit while asking the patient to hold his or her breath briefly.
    d. for unilateral distention while turning the patient's head to one side.

16. Fill in the following blanks:

    S_1 is best heard at the _____ of the heart, whereas S_2 is loudest at the _____ of the heart. S_1 coincides with the pulse in the _____ and coincides with the _____ wave if the patient is on an ECG monitor.

Match column A to column B

Column A

17. _____ tough, fibrous, double-walled sac that surrounds and protects the heart

18. _____ thin layer of endothelial tissue that lines the inner surface of the heart chambers and valves

19. _____ reservoir for holding blood

20. _____ ensures smooth, friction-free movement of the heart muscle

21. _____ muscular pumping chamber

22. _____ muscular wall of the heart

Column B

a. pericardial fluid

b. ventricle

c. endocardium

d. myocardium

e. pericardium

f. atrium

23. Briefly relate the route of a blood cell from the liver to tissue in the body.

24. List the major risk factors for heart disease and stroke identified in the text.

SKILLS LABORATORY/CLINICAL SETTING

You are now ready for the clinical component of the cardiovascular system. The purpose of the clinical component is to practice the regional examination on a peer in the skills laboratory or a patient in the clinical setting and to achieve the following.

Clinical Objectives

1. Demonstrate knowledge of the symptoms related to the cardiovascular system by obtaining a regional health history from a peer or patient.

2. Correctly locate anatomic landmarks on the chest wall of a peer.

3. Using a grease pencil and with peer's permission, outline borders of the heart and label auscultatory areas on a peer's chest wall.

4. Demonstrate correct technique for inspection and palpation of the neck vessels.

5. Demonstrate correct techniques for inspection, palpation, and auscultation of the precordium.

6. Record the history and physical examination findings accurately, reach an assessment of the health state, and develop a plan of care.

Instructions

Gather your equipment. Wash your hands. Clean the stethoscope endpiece with an alcohol wipe. Practice the steps of the examination of the cardiovascular system on a peer or on a patient in the clinical area. Record your findings using the regional write-up sheet that follows. The front of the page is intended as a worksheet; the back of the page is intended for your narrative recording using the SOAP format.

NOTES

REGIONAL WRITE-UP—CARDIOVASCULAR SYSTEM

Date _____

Examiner _____

Patient _____ Age _____ Gender _____

Reason for visit _____

I. Health History

	No	Yes, explain
1. Any **chest pain** or tightness?		
2. Any **shortness of breath**?		
3. Use more than one pillow to sleep?		
4. Do you have a **cough**?		
5. Do you seem to **tire easily**?		
6. Facial skin ever turn blue or ashen?		
7. Any **swelling** of feet or legs?		
8. Awaken at night to urinate?		
9. Any past history of heart disease?		
10. Any family history of heart disease?		

11. Assess cardiac risk factors: _____

II. Physical Examination

A. Carotid arteries

Inspect and palpate

Grade R _____ L _____

(0 = absent, 1+ weak, 2+ normal, 3+ increased, 4+ bounding)

B. Jugular venous system

External jugular veins (circle one): < collapsed supine / meniscus visible at _____ bed elevated

Internal jugular venous pulsations (circle one): < not visible / visible at _____ bed elevated

C. Precordium

Inspect and palpate

1. Skin color and condition _____
2. Chest wall pulsations _____
3. Heave or lift _____
4. Apical impulse in the _____ at _____
   Size _____ Amplitude _____

D. Auscultation

1. Identify anatomic areas where you will listen.
2. Rate and rhythm _____
3. Identify S_1 and S_2 in diagram at right and note any variation.
   Fill in any murmur below:

   S_1 S_2 S_1 S_2

   S_1 _____

   S_2 _____

4. Listen in systole and diastole:
   Extra heart sounds _____
   Systolic murmur _____
   Diastolic murmur _____

REGIONAL WRITE-UP—CARDIOVASCULAR SYSTEM

Summarize your findings using the SOAP format.

Subjective (Reason for seeking care, health history)

Objective (Physical examination findings)   Record findings using diagram

Assessment (Assessment of health state or problem, diagnosis)

Plan (Diagnostic evaluation, follow-up care, patient teaching)

Peripheral Vascular System and Lymphatic System

PURPOSE

This chapter helps you learn the structure and function of the peripheral vascular system and the lymphatic system; locate the peripheral pulse sites; understand the rationale and methods of examination of the peripheral vascular and lymphatic systems; and accurately record the assessment. At the end of this chapter you should be able to perform a complete assessment of the peripheral vascular and lymphatic systems.

READING ASSIGNMENT

Jarvis: *Physical Examination and Health Assessment*, 6th ed., Chapter 20, pp. 499-526.

MEDIA ASSIGNMENT

Jarvis: *Physical Examination and Health Assessment* DVD Series: Cardiovascular System: Peripheral Vascular System and Lymphatic System.

GLOSSARY

Study the following terms after completing the reading assignment. You should be able to cover the definition on the right and define the term out loud.

Allen test . . . . determining the patency of the radial and ulnar arteries by compressing one artery site and observing return of skin color as evidence of patency of the other artery

Aneurysm . . . . defect or sac formed by dilation in artery wall due to atherosclerosis, trauma, or congenital defect

Arrhythmia . . . . variation from the heart's normal rhythm

Arteriosclerosis . . . . thickening and loss of elasticity of the arterial walls

Atherosclerosis . . . . plaques of fatty deposits formed in the inner layer (intima) of the arteries

Bradycardia . . . . slow heart rate, <50 beats per minute in the adult

Bruit . . . . blowing, swooshing sound heard through a stethoscope when an artery is partially occluded

Cyanosis . . . . dusky blue mottling of the skin and mucous membranes due to excessive amount of reduced hemoglobin in the blood

Diastole . . . . the heart's filling phase

Homans' sign . . . . calf pain that occurs when the foot is sharply dorsiflexed (pushed up, toward the knee); may occur with deep vein thrombosis, phlebitis, Achilles tendinitis, or muscle injury

Ischemia . . . . deficiency of arterial blood to a body part due to constriction or obstruction of a blood vessel

Lymphedema . . . . swelling of extremity due to obstructed lymph channel, nonpitting

Lymph nodes . . . . small oval clumps of lymphatic tissue located at grouped intervals along lymphatic vessels

Pitting edema . . . . indentation left after examiner depresses the skin over swollen edematous tissue

Profile sign . . . . viewing the finger from the side to detect early clubbing

Pulse . . . . pressure wave created by each heartbeat, palpable at body sites where the artery lies close to the skin and over a bone

Pulsus alternans . . . . regular rhythm, but force of pulse varies with alternating beats of large and small amplitude

Pulsus bigeminus . . . . irregular rhythm, every other beat is premature; premature beats have weakened amplitude

Pulsus paradoxus . . . . beats have weaker amplitude with respiratory inspiration, stronger with expiration

Systole . . . . the heart's pumping phase

Tachycardia . . . . rapid heart rate, >90 beats per minute in the adult

Thrombophlebitis . . . . inflammation of the vein associated with thrombus formation

Ulcer . . . . open skin lesion extending into dermis with sloughing of necrotic inflammatory tissue

Varicose vein . . . . dilated tortuous veins with incompetent valves

STUDY GUIDE

After completing the reading assignment and the media assignment, you should be able to answer the following questions in the spaces provided.

1. Describe the structure and function of arteries and veins.

2. List the pulse sites accessible to examination.

3. Describe 3 mechanisms that help return venous blood to the heart.

4. Define the term *capacitance vessels,* and explain its significance.

5. List the risk factors for venous stasis.

6. Describe the function of the lymphatic system.

7. Describe the function of the lymph nodes.

8. Name the related organs in the lymphatic system.

9. List the symptom areas to address during history taking of the peripheral vascular system.

10. Fill in the grading scale for assessing the force of an arterial pulse: 0 = _____; 1+_____;
    2+_____; 3+_____

11. List the steps in performing the modified Allen test.

12. List the skin characteristics expected with arterial insufficiency to the lower legs.

13. Compare the characteristics of leg ulcers associated with arterial insufficiency with ulcers with
    venous insufficiency.

14. Fill in the description of the grading scale for pitting edema:

    1+ _____

    2+ _____

    3+ _____

    4+ _____

15. Describe the technique for using the Doppler ultrasonic stethoscope to detect peripheral pulses.

16. Raynaud's phenomenon has associated progressive tricolor changes of the skin from _____ to _____ and then to _____. State the mechanism for each of these color changes.

Fill in the labels indicated on the following arteries and name the pulse sites.

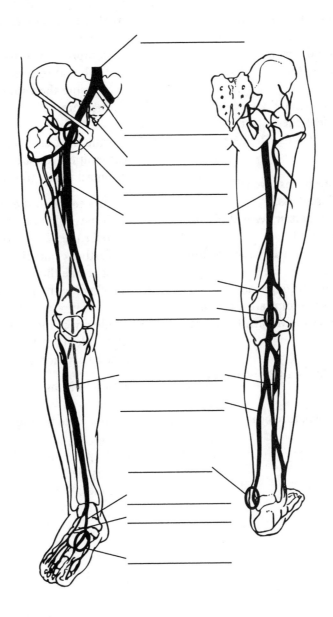

REVIEW QUESTIONS

This test is for you to check your own mastery of the content. Answers are provided in Appendix A.

1. A function of the venous system is:

   a. to hold more blood when blood volume increases.
   b. to conserve fluid and plasma proteins that leak out of the capillaries.
   c. to form a major part of the immune system that defends the body against disease.
   d. to absorb lipids from the intestinal tract.

2. The organs that aid the lymphatic system are:

   a. liver, lymph nodes, and stomach.
   b. pancreas, small intestine, and thymus.
   c. spleen, tonsils, and thymus.
   d. pancreas, spleen, and tonsils.

3. Ms. T. has come for a prenatal visit. She complains of dependent edema, varicosities in the legs, and hemorrhoids. The best response is:

   a. "If these symptoms persist, we will perform an amniocentesis."
   b. "If these symptoms persist, we will discuss having you hospitalized."
   c. "The symptoms are caused by the pressure of the growing uterus on the veins. They are usual conditions of pregnancy."
   d. "At this time, the symptoms are a minor inconvenience. You should learn to accept them."

4. A pulse with an amplitude of 3+ would be considered:

   a. irregular, with 3 premature beats.
   b. increased, full.
   c. normal.
   d. weak.

5. Inspection of a person's right hand reveals a red, swollen area. To further assess for infection, you would palpate the:

   a. cervical node.
   b. axillary node.
   c. epitrochlear node.
   d. inguinal node.

6. To screen for deep vein thrombosis, you would:

   a. measure the circumference of the ankle.
   b. check the temperature with the palm of the hand.
   c. compress the dorsalis pedis pulse, looking for blood return.
   d. measure the widest point with a tape measure.

7. During the examination of the lower extremities, you are unable to palpate the popliteal pulse. You should:

   a. proceed with the examination. It is often impossible to palpate this pulse.
   b. refer the patient to a vascular surgeon for further evaluation.
   c. schedule the patient for a venogram.
   d. schedule the patient for an arteriogram.

8. While reviewing a medical record, a notation of 4+ edema of the right leg is noted. The best description of this type of edema is:

   a. mild pitting, no perceptible swelling of the leg.
   b. moderate pitting, indentation subsides rapidly.
   c. deep pitting, leg looks swollen.
   d. very deep pitting, indentation lasts a long time.

9. The examiner wishes to assess for arterial deficit in the lower extremities. After raising the legs 12 inches off the table and then having the person sit up and dangle the leg, the color should return in:

   a. 5 seconds or less.
   b. 10 seconds or less.
   c. 15 seconds.
   d. 30 seconds.

10. A 54-year-old woman with five children has varicose veins of the lower extremities. Her most characteristic sign is:

    a. reduced arterial circulation.
    b. blanching, deathlike appearance of the extremities on elevation.
    c. loss of hair on feet and toes.
    d. dilated, tortuous superficial bluish vessels.

11. Atrophic skin changes that occur with peripheral arterial insufficiency include:

    a. thin, shiny skin with loss of hair.
    b. brown discoloration.
    c. thick, leathery skin.
    d. slow-healing blisters on the skin.

12. Intermittent claudication is:

    a. muscular pain relieved by exercise.
    b. neurologic pain relieved by exercise.
    c. muscular pain brought on by exercise.
    d. neurologic pain brought on by exercise.

13. A known risk factor for venous ulcer development is:

    a. obesity.
    b. male gender.
    c. history of hypertension.
    d. daily aspirin therapy.

14. Brawny edema is:

    a. acute in onset.
    b. soft.
    c. nonpitting.
    d. associated with diminished pulses.

15. Arteriosclerosis is the:

    a. deposition of fatty plaques on the intima of the arteries.
    b. loss of elasticity of the walls of blood vessels.
    c. loss of lymphatic tissue that occurs in the aging process.
    d. progressive enlargement of the intramuscular calf veins.

16. Raynaud's phenomenon occurs:

    a. when the patient's extremities are exposed to heat and compression.
    b. in hands and feet as a result of exposure to cold, vibration, and stress.
    c. after removal of lymph nodes or damage to lymph nodes and channels.
    d. as a result of leg cramps due to excessive walking or climbing stairs.

SKILLS LABORATORY/CLINICAL SETTING

You are now ready for the clinical component of the peripheral vascular system. The purpose of the clinical component is to practice the regional examination on a peer in the skills laboratory or a patient in the clinical setting and to achieve the following.

Clinical Objectives

1. Demonstrate knowledge of the symptoms related to the peripheral vascular system by obtaining a regional health history from a peer or patient.

2. Demonstrate palpation of peripheral arterial pulses (brachial, radial, femoral, popliteal, posterior tibial, dorsalis pedis) by assessing amplitude and symmetry, noting any signs of arterial insufficiency.

3. Demonstrate inspection and palpation of peripheral veins by noting any signs of venous insufficiency.

4. Demonstrate palpation of lymphatic system by identifying enlargement, clumping, or abnormal firmness of regional lymph nodes.

5. Demonstrate correct technique for performing the following additional tests when indicated: Allen test; manual compression test; Doppler ultrasonic stethoscope; computing the ankle-brachial index (ABI).

6. Record the history and physical examination findings accurately, reach an assessment of the health state, and develop a plan of care.

Instructions

Gather your equipment. Wash your hands. Practice the steps of the examination of the peripheral vascular system on a peer or on a patient in the clinical setting, giving appropriate instructions as you proceed. Record your findings using the regional write-up sheets that follow. The first part is intended as a worksheet; the last page is intended for your narrative summary recording using the SOAP format. Note that the peripheral examination and cardiovascular examination usually are practiced together.

NOTES

REGIONAL WRITE-UP—PERIPHERAL VASCULAR SYSTEM

Date _____

Examiner _____

Patient _____ Age _____ Gender _____

Reason for visit _____

I. **Health History**

	No	Yes, explain
1. Any leg **pain** (cramps)? Where?		
2. Any **skin changes** in arms or legs?		
3. Any sores or **lesions** in arms or legs?		
4. Any **swelling** in the legs?		
5. Any **swollen glands**? Where?		
6. What medications are you taking?		

II. **Physical Examination**

 A. **The Arms**

   Inspect

   Color of skin and nail beds _____

   Symmetry _____

   Lesions _____

   Edema _____

   Clubbing _____

   Palpate

   Temperature _____

   Texture _____

   Capillary refill _____

   Locate and grade pulses (record on back)

   Check epitrochlear lymph nodes _____

   Modified Allen test (if indicated) _____

 B. **The Legs**

   Inspect

   Color _____

   Hair distribution _____

   Venous pattern/varicosities _____

   Size _____

    Swelling/edema _____

    Atrophy _____

    If so, measure calf circumference in cm R _____ L _____

   Skin lesions or ulcers _____

   Palpate

   Temperature _____

   Check Homans' sign _____

   Tenderness _____

   Inguinal lymph nodes _____

   Locate and grade pulses (record on back) _____

   Check pretibial edema (grade if present) _____

   Auscultate for bruit (if indicated) _____

REGIONAL WRITE-UP—PERIPHERAL VASCULAR SYSTEM

	Brachial	Radial	Femoral	Popliteal	D. pedis	P. tibial
R						
L						

0 = absent, 1+ = weak, 2+ = normal, 3+ = full, bounding

C. Additional tests

Manual compression test _____

Check color change: elevate legs, then dangle; color returns in _____ seconds

Doppler ultrasonic stethoscope

   Locate pulse sites

   Ankle-brachial index (ABI)

   _____ ankle systolic pressure

$$\frac{\text{_____}}{\text{_____ arm systolic pressure}} = \text{_____ . _____ or _____ \%}$$

REGIONAL WRITE-UP—PERIPHERAL VASCULAR SYSTEM

Summarize your findings using the SOAP format.

Subjective (Reason for seeking care, health history)

Objective (Physical examination findings)   Record pulses on diagram below

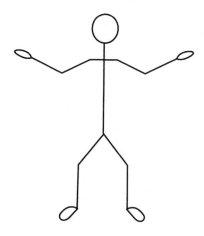

Assessment (Assessment of health state or problem, diagnosis)

Plan (Diagnostic evaluation, follow-up care, teaching)

NOTES

PURPOSE

This chapter helps you learn the structure and function of the abdominal organs; know the location of the abdominal organs; discriminate normal bowel sounds; understand the rationale and methods of examination of the abdomen; and accurately record the assessment. At the end of this chapter you should be able to perform a complete assessment of the abdomen.

READING ASSIGNMENT

Jarvis: *Physical Examination and Health Assessment*, 6th ed., Chapter 21, pp. 527-564.

MEDIA ASSIGNMENT

Jarvis: *Physical Examination and Health Assessment* DVD Series: Abdomen.

GLOSSARY

Study the following terms after completing the reading assignment. You should be able to cover the definition on the right and define the term out loud.

Aneurysm . . . . defect or sac formed by dilation in artery wall due to atherosclerosis, trauma, or congenital defect

Anorexia . . . . loss of appetite for food

Ascites . . . . abnormal accumulation of serous fluid within the peritoneal cavity, associated with congestive heart failure, cirrhosis, cancer, or portal hypertension

Borborygmi . . . . loud, gurgling bowel sounds signaling increased motility or hyperperistalsis, occurs with early bowel obstruction, gastroenteritis, diarrhea

Bruit . . . . blowing, swooshing sound heard through a stethoscope when an artery is partially occluded

Cecum . . . . first or proximal part of large intestine

Cholecystitis . . . . inflammation of the gallbladder

Costal margin . . . . lower border of rib margin formed by the medial edges of the 8th, 9th, and 10th ribs

Costovertebral angle (CVA) . . . angle formed by the 12th rib and the vertebral column on the posterior thorax, overlying the kidney

Diastasis recti . . . . midline longitudinal ridge in the abdomen, a separation of abdominal rectus muscles

Dysphagia . . . . difficulty swallowing

Epigastrium . . . . name of abdominal region between the costal margins

Hepatomegaly . . . . abnormal enlargement of liver

Hernia . . . . abnormal protrusion of bowel through weakening in abdominal musculature

Inguinal ligament . . . . ligament extending from pubic bone to anterior superior iliac spine, forming lower border of abdomen

Linea alba . . . . midline tendinous seam joining the abdominal muscles

Paralytic ileus . . . . complete absence of peristaltic movement that may follow abdominal surgery or complete bowel obstruction

Peritoneal friction rub . . . . rough grating sound heard through the stethoscope over the site of peritoneal inflammation

Peritonitis . . . . inflammation of peritoneum

Pyloric stenosis . . . . congenital narrowing of pyloric sphincter, forming outflow obstruction of stomach

Pyrosis . . . . (heartburn) burning sensation in upper abdomen due to reflux of gastric acid

Rectus abdominis muscles . . . . midline abdominal muscles extending from rib cage to pubic bone

Scaphoid . . . . abnormally sunken abdominal wall as with malnutrition or underweight

Splenomegaly . . . . abnormal enlargement of spleen

Striae . . . . (lineae albicantes) silvery white or pink scar tissue formed by stretching of abdominal skin as with pregnancy or obesity

Suprapubic . . . . name of abdominal region just superior to pubic bone

Tympany . . . . high-pitched, musical, drumlike percussion note heard when percussing over the stomach and intestine

Umbilicus . . . . depression on the abdomen marking site of entry of umbilical cord

Viscera . . . . internal organs

STUDY GUIDE

After completing the reading assignment and the media assignment, you should be able to answer the following questions in the spaces provided.

1. Draw a picture of the borders of the abdomen.
   Draw in the organs.

2. Name the organs that are normally palpable in the abdomen.

3. Describe the proper positioning and preparation of the patient for the examination.

4. State the rationale for performing auscultation of the abdomen before palpation or percussion.

5. Discuss inspection of the abdomen, including findings that should be noted.

6. Describe the procedure for auscultation of bowel sounds.

7. Differentiate the following abdominal sounds: normal, hyperactive, and hypoactive bowel sounds, succession splash, bruit.

8. Identify and give the rationale for each of the percussion notes heard over the abdomen.

   List 4 conditions that may alter normal percussion notes.

9. Describe the procedure for percussing the liver span and the spleen.

10. Describe these maneuvers and discuss their significance: fluid wave test, shifting dullness.

11. Differentiate between light and deep palpation, and explain the purpose of each.

List 2 abnormalities that may be detected by light palpation and 2 detected by deep palpation.

12. Contrast rigidity with voluntary guarding.

13. Contrast visceral pain and somatic (parietal) pain.

14. Describe rebound tenderness.

15. Describe palpation of the liver, spleen, kidney.

16. Distinguish abdominal wall masses from intra-abdominal masses.

17. Describe the procedure and rationale for determining costovertebral angle (CVA) tenderness.

18. Describe the expected examination findings of the abdomen in each of the following conditions:

    Obesity _____

    _____

    Gaseous distention _____

    _____

Tumor _____
_____

Pregnancy _____
_____

Ascites _____
_____

Enlarged liver _____
_____

Enlarged spleen _____
_____

Distended bladder _____
_____

Appendicitis _____
_____

Fill in the labels indicated on the following illustrations.

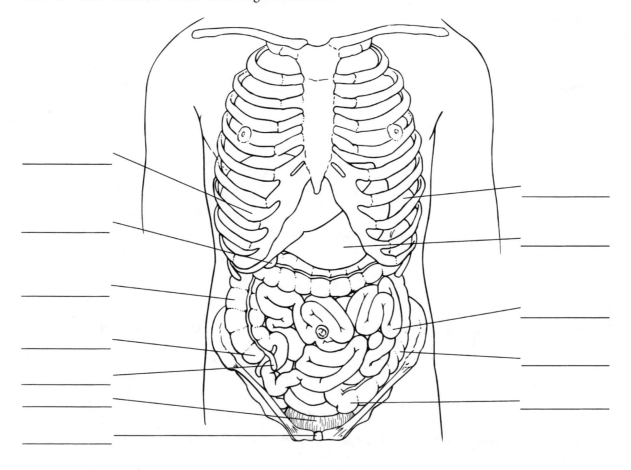

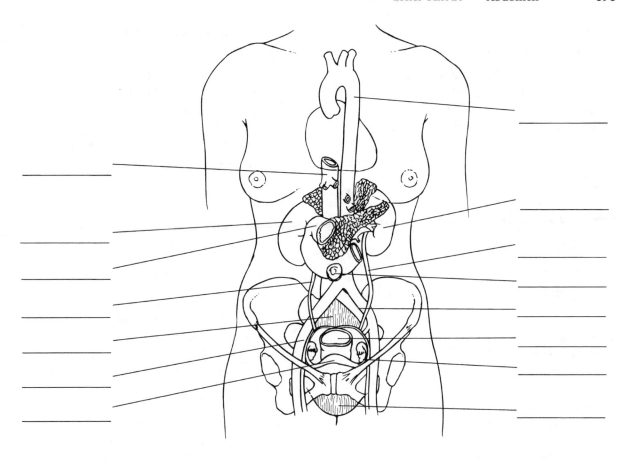

REVIEW QUESTIONS

This test is for you to check your own mastery of the content. Answers are provided in Appendix A.

1. Select the sequence of techniques used during an examination of the abdomen.

   a. percussion, inspection, palpation, auscultation
   b. inspection, palpation, percussion, auscultation
   c. inspection, auscultation, percussion, palpation
   d. auscultation, inspection, palpation, percussion

2. Which of the following may be noted through inspection of the abdomen?

   a. fluid waves and abdominal contour
   b. umbilical eversion and Murphy sign
   c. venous pattern, peristaltic waves, and abdominal contour
   d. peritoneal irritation, general tympany, and peristaltic waves

3. Right upper quadrant tenderness may indicate pathology in the:

   a. liver, pancreas, or ascending colon.
   b. liver and stomach.
   c. sigmoid colon, spleen, or rectum.
   d. appendix or ileocecal valve.

4. Hyperactive bowel sounds are:

   a. high pitched.
   b. rushing.
   c. tinkling.
   d. all of the above.

5. The absence of bowel sounds is established after listening for:

   a. 1 full minute.
   b. 3 full minutes.
   c. 5 full minutes.
   d. none of the above.

6. Auscultation of the abdomen may reveal bruits of the _____ arteries.

   a. aortic, renal, iliac, and femoral
   b. jugular, aortic, carotid, and femoral
   c. pulmonic, aortic, and portal
   d. renal, iliac, internal jugular, and basilic

7. The range of normal liver span in the right midclavicular line in the adult is:

   a. 2-6 cm.
   b. 4-8 cm.
   c. 8-14 cm.
   d. 6-12 cm.

8. The left upper quadrant (LUQ) contains the:

   a. liver.
   b. appendix.
   c. left ovary.
   d. spleen.

9. Striae, which occur when the elastic fibers in the reticular layer of the skin are broken after rapid or prolonged stretching, have a distinct color when of long duration. This color is:

   a. pink.
   b. blue.
   c. purple-blue.
   d. silvery white.

10. Auscultation of the abdomen is begun in the right lower quadrant (RLQ) because:

   a. bowel sounds are always normally present here.
   b. peristalsis through the descending colon is usually active.
   c. this is the location of the pyloric sphincter.
   d. vascular sounds are best heard in this area.

11. A dull percussion note forward of the left midaxillary line is:

   a. normal, an expected finding during splenic percussion.
   b. expected between the 8th and 12th ribs.
   c. found if the examination follows a large meal.
   d. indicative of splenic enlargement.

12. Shifting dullness is a test for:

   a. ascites.
   b. splenic enlargement.
   c. inflammation of the kidney.
   d. hepatomegaly.

13. Tenderness during abdominal palpation is expected when palpating:

   a. the liver edge.
   b. the spleen.
   c. the sigmoid colon.
   d. the kidneys.

14. Murphy sign is best described as:

   a. the pain felt when the hand of the examiner is rapidly removed from an inflamed appendix.
   b. pain felt when taking a deep breath when the examiner's fingers are on the approximate location of the inflamed gallbladder.
   c. a sharp pain felt by the patient when one hand of the examiner is used to thump the other at the costovertebral angle.
   d. not a valid examination technique.

15. A positive Blumberg sign indicates:

   a. a possible aortic aneurysm.
   b. the presence of renal artery stenosis.
   c. an enlarged, nodular liver.
   d. peritoneal inflammation.

16. What is the significance of black stools? Contrast this with the significance of red blood in stools.

SKILLS LABORATORY/CLINICAL SETTING

You are now ready for the clinical component of the abdominal system. The purpose of the clinical component is to practice the regional examination on a peer in the skills laboratory or a patient in the clinical setting and to achieve the following.

Clinical Objectives

1. Demonstrate knowledge of the symptoms related to the abdominal system by obtaining a regional health history from a peer or patient.

2. Demonstrate inspection of the abdomen by assessing skin condition, symmetry, contour, pulsation, umbilicus, nutritional state.

3. Demonstrate auscultation of the abdomen by assessing characteristics of bowel sounds and by screening for bruits.

4. Demonstrate percussion of the abdomen by identifying predominant percussion note, determining liver span, noting borders of spleen.

5. Demonstrate light palpation by assessing muscular resistance, tenderness, any masses.

6. Demonstrate deep palpation by assessing for any masses; the liver, spleen, kidneys, aorta; any CVA or rebound tenderness.

7. Demonstrate correct technique of performing the following additional tests when indicated: inspiratory arrest; iliopsoas muscle test; obturator test.

8. Record the history and physical examination findings accurately, reach an assessment of the health state, and develop a plan of care.

Instructions

Gather your equipment. Wash your hands. Assess the patient's comfort before starting. Practice the steps of the examination on a peer or a patient in the clinical setting, giving appropriate instructions as you proceed. Record your findings using the regional write-up sheets that follow. The front of the page is intended as a worksheet; the back of the page is intended for your narrative summary recording using the SOAP format.

NOTES

REGIONAL WRITE-UP—ABDOMEN

Date _____

Examiner _____

Patient _____ Age _____ Gender _____

Reason for visit _____

I. Health History

	No	Yes, explain
1. Any change in **appetite**? Loss?	_____	_____
2. Any difficulty **swallowing**?	_____	_____
3. Any foods you **cannot tolerate**?	_____	_____
4. Any **abdominal pain**?	_____	_____
5. Any **nausea or vomiting**?	_____	_____
6. How often are **bowel movements**?	_____	_____
7. Any past history of **GI disease**?	_____	_____
8. What **medications** are you taking?	_____	_____

9. Tell me all food you ate in the last **24 hours,** starting with:

breakfast   snack   lunch   snack   dinner   snack

II. Physical Examination

A. Inspection

Contour of abdomen _____

General symmetry _____

Skin color and condition _____

Pulsation or movement _____

Umbilicus _____

State of hydration and nutrition _____

Person's facial expression and position in bed _____

B. Auscultation

Bowel sounds _____

Note any vascular sounds _____

C. Percussion

Percuss in all four quadrants _____

Percuss borders of liver span in R MCL _____ cm

Percuss spleen _____

If suspect ascites, test for fluid wave and shifting dullness _____

D. Palpation

Light palpation in all four quadrants

   Muscle wall _____

   Tenderness _____

   Enlarged organs _____

   Masses _____

Deep palpation in all four quadrants

   Masses _____

   Contour of liver _____

Spleen _____
Kidneys _____
Aorta _____
Rebound tenderness _____
CVA tenderness _____

E. **Additional tests, if indicated**

REGIONAL WRITE-UP—ABDOMEN

Summarize your findings using the SOAP format.

Subjective (Reason for seeking care, health history)

Objective (Physical examination findings)
Record findings on diagram

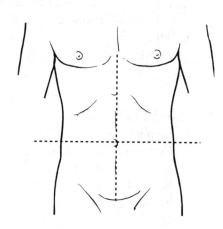

Assessment (Assessment of health state or problem, diagnosis)

Plan (Diagnostic evaluation, follow-up care, teaching)

CHAPTER 22

Musculoskeletal System

PURPOSE

This chapter helps you learn the structure and function of the various joints in the body; know their normal ranges of motion; position the patient comfortably during the examination; understand the rationale and methods of examination of the musculoskeletal system; assess functional ability; and accurately record the assessment. At the end of this chapter you should be able to perform a complete assessment of the musculoskeletal system.

READING ASSIGNMENT

Jarvis: *Physical Examination and Health Assessment,* 6th ed., Chapter 22, pp. 565-620.

MEDIA ASSIGNMENT

Jarvis: *Physical Examination and Health Assessment* DVD Series: Musculoskeletal System.

GLOSSARY

Study the following terms after completing the reading assignment. You should be able to cover the definition on the right and define the term out loud.

Abduction . . . . moving a body part away from an axis or the median line

Adduction . . . . moving a body part toward the center or toward the median line

Ankylosis . . . . immobility, consolidation, and fixation of a joint because of disease, injury, or surgery; most often due to chronic rheumatoid arthritis

Ataxia . . . . inability to perform coordinated movements

Bursa . . . . enclosed sac filled with viscous fluid located in joint areas of potential friction

Circumduction . . . . moving the arm in a circle around the shoulder

Crepitation . . . . dry crackling sound or sensation due to grating of the ends of damaged bone

Dorsal. directed toward or located on the surface

Dupuytren contracture. . . . . . . flexion contracture of the fingers due to chronic hyperplasia of the palmar fascia

Eversion. . . . . moving the sole of the foot outward at the ankle

Extension. . . . . straightening a limb at a joint

Flexion. bending a limb at a joint

Ganglion. . . . . round, cystic, nontender nodule overlying a tendon sheath or joint capsule, usually on dorsum of wrist

Hallux valgus. . . . . lateral or outward deviation of the great toe

Inversion. . . . . moving the sole of the foot inward at the ankle

Kyphosis. . . . . outward or convex curvature of the thoracic spine; hunchback

Ligament. . . . . fibrous band running directly from one bone to another bone that strengthens the joint

Lordosis. . . . . inward or concave curvature of the lumbar spine

Nucleus pulposus. . . . . center of the intervertebral disk

Olecranon process. . . . . bony projection of the ulna at the elbow

Patella. . . . . kneecap

Plantar. surface of the sole of the foot

Pronation. . . . . turning the forearm so that the palm is down

Protraction. . . . . moving a body part forward and parallel to the ground

Range of motion (ROM). . . . . . extent of movement of a joint

Retraction. . . . . moving a body part backward and parallel to the ground

Rheumatoid arthritis. . . . . chronic systemic inflammatory disease of joints and surrounding connective tissue

Sciatica. nerve pain along the course of the sciatic nerve that travels down from the back or thigh through the leg and into the foot

Scoliosis. . . . . S-shaped curvature of the thoracic spine

Supination. . . . . turning the forearm so that the palm is up

Talipes equinovarus. . . . . (clubfoot) congenital deformity of the foot in which it is plantar flexed and inverted

Tendon. strong fibrous cord that attaches a skeletal muscle to a bone

Torticollis. . . . . (wryneck) contraction of the cervical neck muscles, producing torsion of the neck

STUDY GUIDE

After completing the reading assignment and the media assignment, you should be able to answer the following questions in the spaces provided.

1. Differentiate synovial from nonsynovial joints.

2. Draw a section view of the vertebrae and intervertebral disks. Describe the function of the disks.

3. List 4 signs that suggest acute inflammation in a joint.

4. Differentiate the following:

   Dislocation _____

   Subluxation _____

   Contracture _____

   Ankylosis _____

5. Differentiate testing of active range of motion versus passive range of motion.

6. State the expected range of degrees of flexion and extension of the following joints:

   Elbow _____

   Wrist _____

   Fingers (at metacarpophalangeal joints) _____

7. State the expected range of degrees of flexion and extension of the following joints:

   Hip _____

   Knee _____

   Ankle _____

8. Explain the method for measuring leg length.

9. Describe the Ortolani maneuver for checking an infant's hips.

10. State 4 landmarks to note when checking an adolescent for scoliosis.

11. When performing a functional assessment for an older adult, state the common adaptations the aging person makes when attempting these maneuvers:

    Walking _____

    Climbing up stairs _____

    Walking down stairs _____

    Picking up object from floor _____

    Rising up from sitting in chair _____

    _____

    Rising up from lying in bed _____

    _____

12. Describe the symptoms and signs in carpal tunnel syndrome.

    Name and describe 2 techniques of examination for the syndrome.

13. Draw and describe swan neck deformity and boutonnière deformity.

14. Contrast Bouchard's nodes with Heberden's nodes.

15. Contrast syndactyly and polydactyly.

Fill in the labels indicated on the following illustrations.

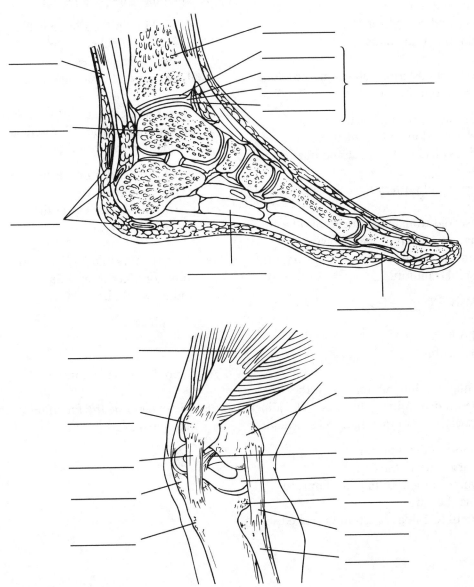

REVIEW QUESTIONS

This test is for you to check your own mastery of the content. Answers are provided in Appendix A.

1. During an assessment of the spine, the patient would be asked to:

   a. adduct and extend.
   b. supinate, evert, and retract.
   c. extend, adduct, invert, and rotate.
   d. flex, extend, abduct, and rotate.

2. Pronation and supination of the hand and forearm are the result of the articulation of the:

   a. scapula and clavicle.
   b. radius and ulna.
   c. patella and condyle of fibula.
   d. femur and acetabulum.

3. Anterior and posterior stability are provided to the knee joint by the:

   a. medial and lateral menisci.
   b. patellar tendon and ligament.
   c. medial collateral ligament and quadriceps muscle.
   d. anterior and posterior cruciate ligaments.

4. A 70-year-old woman has come for a health examination. Which of the following is a common age-related change in the curvature of the spinal column?

   a. lordosis
   b. scoliosis
   c. kyphosis
   d. lateral scoliosis

5. The timing of joint pain may assist the examiner in determining the cause. The joint pain associated with rheumatic fever would:

   a. be worse in the morning.
   b. be worse later in the day.
   c. be worse in the morning but improve during the day.
   d. occur 10 to 14 days after an untreated sore throat.

6. Examination of the shoulder includes four motions. These are:

   a. forward flexion, internal rotation, abduction, and external rotation.
   b. abduction, adduction, pronation, and supination.
   c. circumduction, inversion, eversion, and rotation.
   d. elevation, retraction, protraction, and circumduction.

7. The bulge sign is a test for:

   a. swelling in the suprapatellar pouch.
   b. carpal tunnel syndrome.
   c. Heberden's nodes.
   d. olecranon bursa inflammation.

8. The examiner is going to measure the patient's legs for length discrepancy. The normal finding would be:

   a. no difference in measurements.
   b. 0.5 cm difference.
   c. within 1 cm of each other.
   d. 2 cm difference.

9. A 2-year-old child has been brought to the clinic for a health examination. A common finding would be:

   a. kyphosis.
   b. lordosis.
   c. scoliosis.
   d. no deviation is normal.

10. Briefly describe the functions of the musculoskeletal system.

11. Positive Phalen test and Tinel sign are seen in a patient with:

   a. a torn meniscus.
   b. hallux valgus.
   c. carpal tunnel syndrome.
   d. tennis elbow.

12. When assessing an infant, the examiner completes Ortolani maneuver by:

   a. lifting the newborn and noting a C-shaped curvature of the spine.
   b. gently lifting and abducting the infant's flexed knees while palpating the greater trochanter with the fingers.
   c. comparing the height of the tops of the knees when the knees are flexed up.
   d. palpating the length of the clavicles.

Match column A to column B.

Column A—Movement

13. _____ flexion

14. _____ extension

15. _____ abduction

16. _____ adduction

17. _____ pronation

18. _____ supination

19. _____ circumduction

20. _____ inversion

21. _____ eversion

22. _____ rotation

23. _____ protraction

24. _____ retraction

25. _____ elevation

26. _____ depression

Column B—Description

a. turning the forearm so that the palm is up

b. bending a limb at a joint

c. lowering a body part

d. turning the forearm so that the palm is down

e. straightening a limb at a joint

f. raising a body part

g. moving a limb away from the midline of the body

h. moving a body part backward and parallel to the ground

i. moving a limb toward the midline of the body

j. moving the arm in a circle around the shoulder

k. moving the sole of the foot outward at the ankle

l. moving a body part forward and parallel to the ground

m. moving the sole of the foot inward at the ankle

n. moving the head around a central axis

SKILLS LABORATORY/CLINICAL SETTING

You are now ready for the clinical component of the musculoskeletal system. The purpose of the clinical component is to practice the regional examination on a peer in the skills laboratory or a patient in the clinical setting and to achieve the following.

Clinical Objectives

1. Demonstrate knowledge of the symptoms related to the musculoskeletal system by obtaining a regional health history from a peer or patient.

2. Demonstrate inspection and palpation of the musculoskeletal system by assessing the muscles, bones, and joints for size, symmetry, swelling, nodules, deformities, atrophy, and active range of motion.

3. Assess the person's ability to carry out functional activities of daily living.

4. Record the history and physical examination findings accurately, reach an assessment about the health state, and develop a plan of care.

Instructions

Gather your equipment. Wash your hands. Practice the steps of the examination on a peer or a patient in the clinical setting, giving appropriate instructions as you proceed and maintaining the safety of the person during movement. Record your findings using the regional write-up sheet that follows. The first section is intended as a worksheet; the last page is intended for your narrative summary recording using the SOAP format.

Note the student performance checklist that follows the regional write-up sheet. It lists the essential behaviors you should display as an examiner, and it may be used by your clinical instructor to evaluate your clinical musculoskeletal examination.

NOTES

REGIONAL WRITE-UP—MUSCULOSKELETAL SYSTEM

Date _____

Examiner _____

Patient _____ Age _____ Gender _____

Reason for visit _____

I. Health History

	No	Yes, explain
1. Any **pain** in the joints?	_____	_____
2. Any **stiffness** in the joints?	_____	
3. Any **swelling, heat, redness** in joints?	_____	
4. Any **limitation of movement**?	_____	
5. Any **muscle pain** or cramping?	_____	
6. Any **deformity** of bone or joint?	_____	
7. Any **accidents or trauma** to bones?	_____	
8. Ever had **back pain**?	_____	
9. Any problems with the activities of daily living: bathing, toileting, dressing, grooming, eating, mobility, communicating?	_____	

II. Physical Examination

A. Cervical spine

1. Inspect size, contour _____ Mass or deformity _____
2. Palpate for temperature _____ Pain _____
   Swelling or mass _____
3. Active range of motion
   Flexion _____ Extension _____
   Lateral bending right _____ Left _____
   Right rotation _____ Left _____

B. Shoulders

1. Inspect size, contour _____ Color, swelling _____
   Mass or deformity _____
2. Palpate for temperature _____ Pain _____
   Swelling or mass _____
3. Active range of motion
   Flexion _____ Extension _____
   Abduction _____ Adduction _____
   Internal rotation _____ External rotation _____

C. Elbows

1. Inspect for size, contour _____ Color, swelling _____
   Mass or deformity _____
2. Palpate for temperature _____ Pain _____
   Swelling or mass _____
3. Active range of motion
   Flexion _____ Extension _____
   Pronation _____ Supination _____

D. Wrists and hands

1. Inspect for size, contour _____ Color, swelling _____
   Mass or deformity _____
2. Palpate for temperature _____ Pain _____
   Swelling or mass _____
3. Active range of motion
   Wrist extension _____ Flexion _____
   Finger extension _____ Flexion _____
   Ulnar deviation _____ Radial deviation _____
   Fingers spread _____ Make fist _____
   Touch thumb to each finger _____

E. Hips

1. Inspect for size, contour _____ Color, swelling _____
   Mass or deformity _____
2. Palpate for temperature _____ Pain _____
   Swelling or mass _____
3. Active range of motion
   Extension _____ Flexion _____
   External rotation _____ Internal rotation _____
   Abduction _____ Adduction _____

F. Knees

1. Inspect size, contour _____ Color, swelling _____
   Mass or deformity _____
2. Palpate for temperature _____ Pain _____
   Swelling or mass _____
3. Active range of motion
   Flexion _____ Extension _____
   Walk _____ Shallow knee bend _____

G. Ankles and feet

1. Inspect for size, contour _____ Color, swelling _____
   Mass or deformity _____
2. Palpate for temperature _____ Pain _____
   Swelling or mass _____
3. Active range of motion
   Dorsiflexion _____ Plantar flexion _____
   Inversion _____ Eversion _____

H. Spine

   1. Inspect for straight spinous processes _____

       Equal horizontal positions for shoulders, scapulae, iliac crests, gluteal folds _____

       Equal spaces between arms and lateral thorax _____

       Knees and feet align with trunk, point forward _____

       From side, note curvature: cervical, thoracic, lumbar _____

   2. Palpate spinous processes

   3. Active range of motion

       Flexion _____ Extension _____

       Lateral bending right _____ Left _____

       Rotation right _____ Left _____

I. Functional assessment (if indicated)

       Walk (with shoes on)

       Climb up stairs

       Walk down stairs

       Pick up object from floor

       Rise up from sitting in chair

       Rise up from lying in bed

REGIONAL WRITE-UP—MUSCULOSKELETAL SYSTEM

Summarize your findings using the SOAP format.

Subjective (Reason for seeking care, health history)

Objective (Physical examination findings)

Assessment (Assessment of health state or problem, diagnosis)

Plan (Diagnostic evaluation, follow-up care, patient teaching)

STUDENT COMPETENCY CHECKLIST

MUSCULOSKELETAL SYSTEM—ESSENTIAL BEHAVIORS

	Yes	No	Comments
Obtain relevant history, functional and self-care assessments			
Gather equipment:			
Tape measure			
Skin marking pen			
Light if needed			
Provide privacy			
Wash hands			
Observe for symmetry			
Inspect each joint for:			
Size			
Contour			
Range of motion/limitation			
Inspect skin and tissue over joints for:			
Color			
Swelling			
Masses			
Deformity			
Palpate each joint for:			
Heat			
Tenderness			
Swelling			
Masses			
Test ROM			
Grade muscle strength			
Record findings including notations regarding specific joints:			
Temporomandibular			
Cervical spine			
Shoulders			
Elbow			

continued

	Yes	No	Comments
Wrist			
Hand			
Hip			
Knee:			
Ballottement test			
McMurray test			
Ankle			
Foot			
Document findings			

NOTES

CHAPTER 23

Neurologic System

PURPOSE

This chapter helps you learn the structure and function of the components of the neurologic system including the cranial nerves, cerebellar system, motor system, sensory system, and reflexes; understand the rationale and methods of examination of the neurologic system; and accurately record the assessment. Together with the mental status assessment presented in Chapter 6, you should be able to perform a complete assessment of the neurologic system at the end of this chapter.

READING ASSIGNMENT

Jarvis: *Physical Examination and Health Assessment,* 6th ed., Chapter 23, pp. 621-678.

MEDIA ASSIGNMENT

Jarvis: *Physical Examination and Health Assessment* DVD Series: Neurologic: Cranial Nerves and Sensory System; Neurologic: Motor System and Reflexes.

GLOSSARY

Study the following terms after completing the reading assignment. You should be able to cover the definition on the right and define the term out loud.

Agnosia . . . . loss of ability to recognize importance of sensory impressions

Agraphia . . . . loss of ability to express thoughts in writing

Amnesia . . . . loss of memory

Analgesia . . . . loss of pain sensation

Aphasia . . . . loss of power of expression by speech, writing, or signs, or loss of comprehension of spoken or written language

Apraxia . . . . loss of ability to perform purposeful movements in the absence of sensory or motor damage (e.g., inability to use objects correctly)

Ataxia . . . . inability to perform coordinated movements

Athetosis . . . . bizarre, slow, twisting, writhing movement, resembling a snake or worm

Chorea . . . . sudden, rapid, jerky, purposeless movement involving limbs, trunk, or face

Clonus . . . . rapidly alternating involuntary contraction and relaxation of a muscle in response to sudden stretch

Coma . . . . state of profound unconsciousness from which person cannot be aroused

Decerebrate rigidity . . . . arms stiffly extended, adducted, internally rotated; legs stiffly extended, plantar flexed

Decorticate rigidity . . . . arms adducted and flexed, wrists and fingers flexed; legs extended, internally rotated, plantar flexed

Dysarthria . . . . imperfect articulation of speech due to problems of muscular control resulting from central or peripheral nervous system damage

Dysphasia . . . . impairment in speech consisting of lack of coordination and inability to arrange words in their proper order

Extinction . . . . disappearance of conditioned response

Fasciculation . . . . rapid continuous twitching of resting muscle without movement of limb

Flaccidity . . . . loss of muscle tone, limp

Graphesthesia . . . . ability to "read" a number by having it traced on the skin

Hemiplegia . . . . loss of motor power (paralysis) on one side of the body, usually caused by a stroke; paralysis occurs on the side opposite the lesion

Lower motor neuron . . . . motor neuron in the peripheral nervous system with its nerve fiber extending out to the muscle and only its cell body in the central nervous system

Myoclonus . . . . rapid sudden jerk of a muscle

Nuchal rigidity . . . . stiffness in cervical neck area

Nystagmus . . . . back-and-forth oscillation of the eyes

Opisthotonos . . . . prolonged arching of back, with head and heels bent backward, and meningeal irritation

Paralysis . . . . decreased or loss of motor function due to problem with motor nerve or muscle fibers

Paraplegia . . . . impairment or loss of motor and/or sensory function in the lower half of the body

Paresthesia . . . . abnormal sensation (i.e., burning, numbness, tingling, prickling, crawling skin sensation)

Point localization . . . . ability of the person to discriminate exactly where on the body the skin has been touched

Proprioception . . . . sensory information concerning body movements and position of the body in space

Spasticity . . . . continuous resistance to stretching by a muscle due to abnormally increased tension, with increased deep tendon reflexes

Stereognosis . . . . ability to recognize objects by feeling their forms, sizes, and weights while the eyes are closed

Jarvis, Carolyn: PHYSICAL EXAMINATION AND HEALTH ASSESSMENT: Sixth Edition,
Student Laboratory Manual. Copyright © 2012, 2008, 2004, 2000, 1996 by Saunders, an imprint of Elsevier Inc. All rights reserved.

Tic . . . . repetitive twitching of a muscle group at inappropriate times (e.g., wink, grimace)

Tremor . . . . involuntary contraction of opposing muscle groups resulting in rhythmic movement of one or more joints

Two-point discrimination . . . . . ability to distinguish the separation of two simultaneous pinpricks on the skin

Upper motor neuron . . . . nerve located entirely within the central nervous system

STUDY GUIDE

After completing the reading assignment and the media assignment, you should be able to answer the following questions in the spaces provided.

1. List the major function(s) of the following components of the central nervous system:

   Cerebral cortex—frontal lobe _____

   Cerebral cortex—parietal lobe _____

   Cerebral cortex—temporal lobe _____

   Cerebral cortex—Wernicke's area _____

   Cerebral cortex—Broca's area _____

   Basal ganglia _____

   _____

   Thalamus _____

   Hypothalamus _____

   _____

   Cerebellum _____

   Midbrain _____

   Pons _____

   Medulla _____

   Spinal cord _____

2. List the primary sensations mediated by the 2 major sensory pathways of the CNS.

3. Describe 3 major motor pathways in the CNS including the type of movements mediated by each.

4. Differentiate an upper motor neuron from a lower motor neuron.

5. List the 5 components of a deep tendon reflex arc.

6. List the major symptom areas to assess when collecting a health history for the neurologic system.

7. List the method of testing for each of the 12 cranial nerves.

8. List and describe 3 tests of cerebellar function.

9. Describe the method of testing the sensory system for pain, temperature, touch, vibration, and position.

10. Define the 4-point grading scale for deep tendon reflexes.

11. State the vertebral level whose intactness is assessed when eliciting each of these reflexes:

Biceps reflex _____   Quadriceps reflex _____

Triceps reflex _____   Achilles reflex _____

Brachioradialis reflex _____

12. List the components of the neurologic recheck examination that are performed routinely on hospitalized persons being monitored for neurologic deficit.

13. List the 3 areas of assessment on the Glasgow Coma Scale.

14. Describe the gait patterns of the following abnormal gaits:

Spastic hemiparesis _____

Cerebellar ataxia _____

Parkinsonian _____

_____

Scissors _____

Steppage _____

Waddling _____

15. State the type of reflex response you would expect to see with an upper motor neuron lesion versus a lower motor neuron lesion.

16. Describe the method of testing the type of reflexes that are also termed *frontal release signs*.

NOTES

Fill in the labels indicated on the following illustrations.

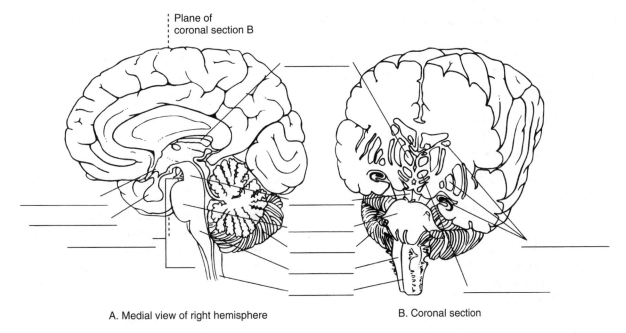

Plane of
coronal section B

A. Medial view of right hemisphere

B. Coronal section

CONTENTS OF THE CENTRAL NERVOUS SYSTEM

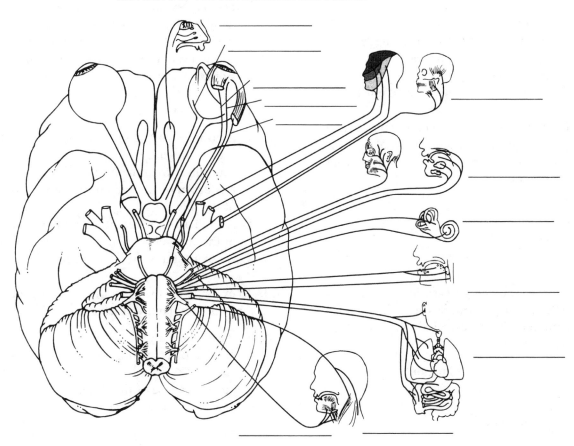

Fill in the name of each cranial nerve, and then write S (sensory), M (motor), or MX (mixed).

REVIEW QUESTIONS

This test is for you to check your own mastery of the content. The answers are provided in Appendix A.

1. The medical record indicates that a person has an injury to Broca's area. When meeting this person you expect:

   a. difficulty speaking.
   b. receptive aphasia.
   c. visual disturbances.
   d. emotional lability.

2. The control of body temperature is located in:

   a. Wernicke's area.
   b. the thalamus.
   c. the cerebellum.
   d. the hypothalamus.

3. To test for stereognosis, you would:

   a. have the person close his or her eyes, and then raise the person's arm and ask the person to describe its location.
   b. touch the person with a tuning fork.
   c. place a coin in the person's hand and ask him or her to identify it.
   d. touch the person with a cold object.

4. During the examination of an infant, use a cotton-tipped applicator to stimulate the anal sphincter. The absence of a response suggests a lesion of:

   a. L2.
   b. T12.
   c. S2.
   d. C5.

5. During a neurologic examination, the tendon reflex fails to appear. Before striking the tendon again, the examiner might use the technique of:

   a. two-point discrimination.
   b. reinforcement.
   c. vibration.
   d. graphesthesia.

6. Cerebellar function is assessed by which of the following tests?

   a. muscle size and strength
   b. cranial nerve examination
   c. coordination—hop on one foot
   d. spinothalamic test

7. To elicit a Babinski reflex:

   a. gently tap the Achilles tendon.
   b. stroke the lateral aspect of the sole of the foot from heel to the ball.
   c. present a noxious odor to the person.
   d. observe the person walking heel to toe.

8. A positive Babinski sign is:

   a. dorsiflexion of the big toe and fanning of all toes.
   b. plantar flexion of the big toe with a fanning of all toes.
   c. the expected response in healthy adults.
   d. withdrawal of the stimulated extremity from the stimulus.

9. The cremasteric response:

   a. is positive when disease of the pyramidal tract is present.
   b. is positive when the ipsilateral testicle elevates upon stroking of the inner aspect of the thigh.
   c. is a reflex of the receptors in the muscles of the abdomen.
   d. is not a valid neurologic examination.

10. To examine for the function of the trigeminal nerve in an infant, you would:

    a. startle the baby.
    b. hold an object within the child's line of vision.
    c. pinch the nose of the child.
    d. offer the baby a bottle.

11. Senile tremors may resemble parkinsonism, except that senile tremors do not include:

    a. nodding the head as if responding yes or no.
    b. rigidity and weakness of voluntary movement.
    c. tremor of the hands.
    d. tongue protrusion.

12. People who have Parkinson disease usually have which of the following characteristic styles of speech?

    a. a garbled manner
    b. loud, urgent
    c. slow, monotonous
    d. word confusion

13. The Glasgow Coma Scale (GCS) is divided into three areas. They include:

    a. pupillary response, a reflex test, and assessing pain.
    b. eye opening, motor response to stimuli, and verbal response.
    c. response to fine touch, stereognosis, and sense of position.
    d. orientation, rapid alternating movements, and the Romberg test.

14. The Landau reflex in the infant is seen when:

    a. the head is held and then flops forward as the baby is pulled to a sitting position by holding the wrists.
    b. the toes curl down tightly in response to touch on the ball of the baby's foot.
    c. the infant attempts to place his foot on the table while being held with the top of the foot touching the underside of the table.
    d. the baby raises the head and arches the back, as in a swan dive.

Match column A to column B.

Column A—Cranial nerve

15. _____ Olfactory

16. _____ Optic

17. _____ Oculomotor

18. _____ Trochlear

19. _____ Trigeminal

20. _____ Abducens

21. _____ Facial

22. _____ Acoustic

23. _____ Glossopharyngeal

24. _____ Vagus

25. _____ Spinal

26. _____ Hypoglossal

Column B—Function

a. movement of the tongue

b. vision

c. lateral movement of the eyes

d. hearing and equilibrium

e. talking, swallowing, and sensory information from pharynx and carotid sinus

f. smell

g. extraocular movement, pupil constriction, down and inward movement of the eye

h. mastication and sensation of face, scalp, cornea

i. phonation, swallowing, taste posterior third of tongue

j. movement of trapezius and sternomastoid muscles

k. down and inward movement of the eye

l. taste anterior two thirds of tongue, close eyes

Jarvis, Carolyn: PHYSICAL EXAMINATION AND HEALTH ASSESSMENT: Sixth Edition,
Student Laboratory Manual. Copyright © 2012, 2008, 2004, 2000, 1996 by Saunders, an imprint of Elsevier Inc. All rights reserved.

SKILLS LABORATORY/CLINICAL SETTING

You are now ready for the clinical component of the neurologic system. The purpose of the clinical component is to practice the regional examination on a peer in the skills laboratory or a patient in the clinical setting and to achieve the following.

Clinical Objectives

1. Demonstrate knowledge of the symptoms related to the neurologic system by obtaining a regional health history from a peer or patient.

2. Demonstrate examination of the neurologic system by assessing the cranial nerves, cerebellar function, sensory system, motor system, and deep tendon reflexes.

3. Record the history and physical examination findings accurately, reach an assessment of the health state, and develop a plan of care.

Instructions

Gather all equipment for a complete neurologic examination. Wash your hands. Practice the steps of the examination on a peer or a patient in the clinical setting, giving appropriate instructions as you proceed. Record your findings using the regional write-up sheet that follows. The first section is intended as a worksheet; the last page is intended for your narrative summary recording using the SOAP format.

NOTES

REGIONAL WRITE-UP—NEUROLOGIC SYSTEM

Date _____

Examiner _____

Patient _____ Age _____ Gender _____

Reason for visit _____

I. Health History

	No	Yes, explain
1. Any unusually frequent or unusually severe **headaches**?	_____	_____
2. Ever had any **head injury**?	_____	_____
3. Ever feel **dizziness**?	_____	_____
4. Ever had any **convulsions**?	_____	_____
5. Any **tremors** in hands or face?	_____	_____
6. Any **weakness** in any body part?	_____	_____
7. Any problem with **coordination**?	_____	_____
8. Any **numbness or tingling**?	_____	_____
9. Any problem **swallowing**?	_____	_____
10. Any problem **speaking**?	_____	_____
11. Past history of stroke, spinal cord injury, meningitis, congenital defect, alcoholism?	_____	_____
12. Any environmental/occupational hazards (e.g., insecticides)?	_____	_____

II. Physical Examination
A. Cranial nerves

I _____

II _____

III, IV, VI _____

V _____

VII _____

VIII _____

IX, X _____

XI _____

XII _____

B. Motor system

1. Muscles
   Size, strength, tone _____

   Involuntary movements _____

2. Cerebellar function
   Gait _____

   Romberg test _____

   Rapid alternative movements _____

   Finger-to-finger test _____

   Finger-to-nose test _____

   Heel-to-shin test _____

C. Sensory system

1. Spinothalamic tract
   Pain _____

   Temperature _____

   Light touch _____

2. Posterior column tract
   Vibration _____

   Position (kinesthesia) _____

   Tactile discrimination _____

   Stereognosis _____

   Graphesthesia _____

   Two-point discrimination _____

D. Reflexes

	Bi	Tri	BR	P	A	PL(↑/↓)	Abd	Cre	Bab
R									
L									

0 = absent, 1+ = hypoactive, 2+ = normal, 3+ = hyperactive, 4+ = hyperactive with clonus, ↑ dorsiflexion, ↓ plantar flexion.

REGIONAL WRITE-UP—NEUROLOGIC SYSTEM

Summarize your findings using the SOAP format.

Subjective (Reason for seeking care, health history)

Objective (Physical examination findings)

Record reflexes on diagram below

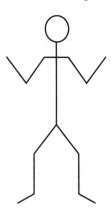

Assessment (Assessment of health state or problem, diagnosis)

Plan (Diagnostic evaluation, follow-up care, patient teaching)

NOTES

PURPOSE

This chapter helps you learn the structure and function of the male genitalia; learn the methods of inspection and palpation of these structures; and record the assessment accurately.

READING ASSIGNMENT

Jarvis: *Physical Examination and Health Assessment*, 6th ed., Chapter 24, pp. 679-708.

MEDIA ASSIGNMENT

Jarvis: *Physical Examination and Health Assessment* DVD Series: Male Genitalia.

GLOSSARY

Study the following terms after completing the reading assignment. You should be able to cover the definition on the right and define the term out loud.

Chancre . . . . red, round, superficial ulcer with a yellowish serous discharge that is a sign of syphilis

Condylomata acuminata . . . . . . soft, pointed, fleshy papules that occur on the genitalia and are caused by the human papillomavirus (HPV)

Cryptorchidism . . . . undescended testes

Cystitis . . . . inflammation of the urinary bladder

Epididymis . . . . structure composed of coiled ducts located over the superior and posterior surface of the testes, which stores sperm

Epispadias . . . . congenital defect in which urethra opens on the dorsal (upper) side of penis instead of at the tip

Hernia . . . . weak spot in abdominal muscle wall (usually in area of inguinal canal or femoral canal) through which a loop of bowel may protrude

Herpes genitalis . . . . a sexually transmitted infection characterized by clusters of small painful vesicles, caused by a virus

Hydrocele . . . . cystic fluid in tunica vaginalis surrounding testis

Hypospadias . . . . congenital defect in which urethra opens on the ventral (under) side of penis rather than at the tip

Orchitis . . . . acute inflammation of testis, usually associated with mumps

Paraphimosis . . . . foreskin is retracted and fixed behind the glans penis

Peyronie disease . . . . nontender, hard plaques on the surface of penis, associated with painful bending of penis during erection

Phimosis . . . . foreskin is advanced and tightly fixed over the glans penis

Prepuce . . . . (foreskin) the hood or flap of skin over the glans penis that often is surgically removed after birth by circumcision

Priapism . . . . prolonged, painful erection of penis without sexual desire

Spermatic cord . . . . collection of vas deferens, blood vessels, lymphatics, and nerves that ascends along the testis and through the inguinal canal into the abdomen

Spermatocele . . . . retention cyst in epididymis filled with milky fluid that contains sperm

Torsion . . . . sudden twisting of spermatic cord; a surgical emergency

Varicocele . . . . dilated tortuous varicose veins in the spermatic cord

Vas deferens . . . . duct carrying sperm from the epididymis through the abdomen and then into the urethra

STUDY GUIDE

After completing the reading assignment and the media assignment, you should be able to answer the following questions in the spaces provided.

1. Describe the function of the cremaster muscle.

2. Identify the structures that provide transport of sperm.

3. Describe the significance of the inguinal canal and the femoral canal.

4. List the pros and cons of circumcision of the male newborn.

5. Discuss ways of creating an environment that will provide psychological comfort for the man and the examiner during examination of male genitalia.

6. List teaching points to include with the teaching of testicular self-examination.

7. List laboratory tests to assess urinary function.

8. Discuss the rationale for making certain that testes have descended in the male infant.

9. Contrast phimosis with paraphimosis; hypospadias with epispadias.

10. Describe the following lesions of the penis and genital area

Tinea cruris

Herpes simplex type 2

Syphilitic chancre

Penile warts (condylomata acuminate, HPV)

11. Contrast the physical appearance and clinical significance of these scrotal lumps:

Epididymitis

Varicocele

Spermatocele

Testicular tumor

Hydrocele

12. Contrast the anatomic course and the clinical significance of these hernias:

Indirect inguinal

Direct inguinal

Femoral

Fill in the labels indicated on the following illustrations.

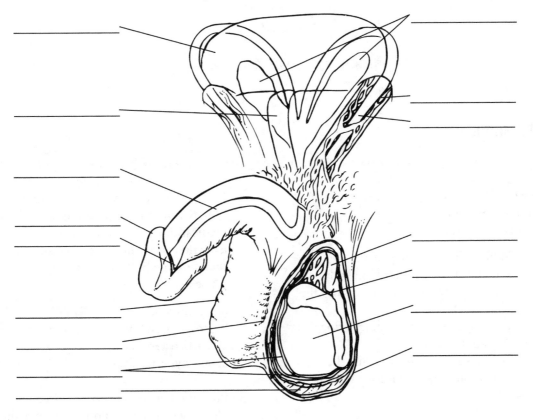

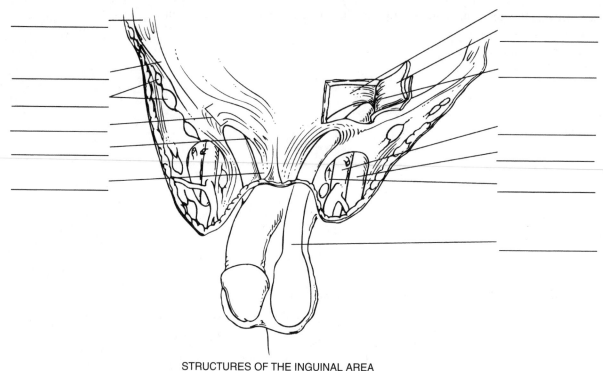

STRUCTURES OF THE INGUINAL AREA

REVIEW QUESTIONS

This test is for you to check your own mastery of the content. Answers are provided in Appendix A.

1. The examiner is going to inspect and palpate for a hernia. During this examination, the man is instructed to:

   a. hold his breath during palpation.
   b. cough after the examiner has gently inserted the examination finger into the rectum.
   c. bear down when the examiner's finger is at the inguinal canal.
   d. relax in a supine position while the examination finger is inserted into the canal.

2. During examination of the scrotum, a normal finding would be:

   a. The left testicle is firmer to palpation than the right.
   b. The left testicle is larger than the right.
   c. The left testicle hangs lower than the right.
   d. The left testicle is more tender to palpation than the right.

3. H.T. has come to the clinic for a follow-up visit. Six months ago, he was started on a new medication. The class of medication is most likely to cause impotence as a side effect; therefore medication classes explored by the nurse are:

   a. antipyretics.
   b. bronchodilators.
   c. corticosteroids.
   d. antihypertensives.

4. Prostatic hypertrophy occurs frequently in older men. The symptoms that may indicate this problem are:

   a. polyuria and urgency.
   b. dysuria and oliguria.
   c. straining, loss of force, and sense of residual urine.
   d. foul-smelling urine and dysuria.

5. A 64-year-old man has come for a health examination. A normal age-related change in the scrotum would be:

   a. testicular atrophy.
   b. testicular hypertrophy.
   c. pendulous scrotum.
   d. increase in scrotal rugae.

6. During palpation of the testes, the normal finding would be:

   a. firm to hard, and rough.
   b. nodular.
   c. 2 to 3 cm long by 2 cm wide and firm.
   d. firm, rubbery, and smooth.

7. A 20-year-old man has indicated that he does not perform testicular self-examination. One of the facts that should be shared with him is that testicular cancer, though rare, does occur in men ages:

   a. younger than 15 years.
   b. 15 to 34 years.
   c. 35 to 55 years.
   d. 55 years and older.

8. During the examination of a full-term newborn male, a finding requiring investigation would be:

   a. absent testes.
   b. meatus centered at the tip of the penis.
   c. wrinkled scrotum.
   d. penis 2 to 3 cm in length.

9. During transillumination of a scrotum, you note a nontender mass that transilluminates with a red glow. This finding is suggestive of:

   a. scrotal hernia.
   b. scrotal edema.
   c. orchitis.
   d. hydrocele.

10. How sensitive to pressure are normal testes?

    a. somewhat
    b. not at all
    c. left is more sensitive than right
    d. only when inflammation is present

11. The congenital displacement of the urethral meatus to the inferior surface of the penis is:

    a. hypospadias.
    b. epispadias.
    c. hypoesthesia.
    d. hypophysis.

12. An adhesion of the prepuce to the head of the penis, making it impossible to retract, is:

    a. paraphimosis.
    b. phimosis.
    c. smegma.
    d. dyschezia.

13. The first physical sign associated with puberty in boys is:

    a. height spurt.
    b. penis lengthening.
    c. sperm production.
    d. pubic hair development.
    e. testes enlargement.

14. Write a narrative account of an assessment of male genitalia with healthy findings.

15. In the aging male, when does infertility occur?

    a. At age 60, with the sudden decline in sperm production.
    b. At approximately age 55 to 60, when testosterone levels are lower.
    c. When the male is not longer able to achieve an erection.
    d. There is no specific age; men may be fertile into their 80s and 90s.

16. A patient has soft, moist, fleshy, painless papules around the anus. The examiner suspects this condition is:

    a. HSV-2.
    b. HPV.
    c. gonorrhea.
    d. Peyronie disease.

SKILLS LABORATORY/CLINICAL SETTING

You are now ready for the clinical component of the male genitalia examination. Because of the need to maintain personal privacy, it is likely you will not practice this examination on a classmate. Your practice likely will be with a teaching mannequin in the skills laboratory or with a male in the clinical setting. Before you proceed, discuss the feelings that may be experienced by the man and the examiner and methods to increase the comfort of both. Make sure you have discussed the steps of the examination with your instructor before examining a patient.

Clinical Objectives

1. Demonstrate knowledge of the signs and symptoms related to the male genitalia by obtaining a pertinent health history.

2. Inspect and palpate the penis and scrotum.

3. Palpate the inguinal region for hernia.

4. Teach testicular self-examination.

5. Record the history and physical examination findings accurately, reach an assessment of the health state, and develop a plan of care.

Instructions

Prepare the examination setting, and gather your equipment. Wash your hands; wear gloves during the examination. Practice the steps of the examination on a male in the clinical setting, giving appropriate instructions as you proceed. Record your findings using the regional write-up sheet that follows. The front of the page is intended as a worksheet; the back of the page is intended for your narrative summary recording using the SOAP format.

Note the student performance checklist that follows the regional write-up sheet. It lists the essential behaviors you should display as an examiner, and it may be used by your clinical instructor to evaluate your clinical teaching of testicular self-examination.

REGIONAL WRITE-UP—MALE GENITOURINARY SYSTEM

Date _____

Examiner _____

Patient _____ Age _____ Gender _____

Reason for visit _____

I. Health History

	No	Yes, explain
1. Any urinary **frequency, urgency,** or awakening during night to urinate?		
2. Any **pain** or **burning** with urinating?		
3. Any **trouble starting urine stream**?		
4. Urine **color cloudy** or **foul-smelling**?		
Red-tinged or **bloody**?		
5. Any **problem controlling your urine**?		
6. Any **pain** or **sores** on penis?		
7. Any **lump** in testicles or scrotum?		
Do you perform testicular self-examination?		
8. In relationship now involving intercourse?		
Use a contraceptive? Which one?		
9. Any contact with partner who has sexually transmitted infection?		

II. Physical Examination

A. Inspect and palpate penis
Skin condition _____
Glans _____
Urethral meatus _____
Shaft _____

B. Inspect and palpate scrotum
Skin condition _____
Testes _____
Spermatic cord _____
Transillumination (if indicated) _____

C. Inspect and palpate for hernia
Inguinal canal _____
Femoral area _____

D. Palpate inguinal lymph nodes _____

E. Teach testicular self-examination

REGIONAL WRITE-UP—MALE GENITOURINARY SYSTEM

Summarize your findings using the SOAP format.

Subjective (Reason for seeking care, health history)

Objective (Physical examination findings)

Assessment (Assessment of health state or problem, diagnosis)

Plan (Diagnostic evaluation, follow-up care, patient teaching)

STUDENT COMPETENCY CHECKLIST

TEACHING TESTICULAR SELF-EXAMINATION (TSE)

	S	U	Comments
I. Cognitive 1. Explain: a. why testicles are examined			
b. who			
c. frequency			
2. Describe the technique			
II. Performance			
1. Explains to male need for TSE			
2. Instructs male on technique of TSE by:			
a. describing method of palpating testicles			
b. describing normal findings			
c. describing abnormal findings to look for			
3. Instructs male to report unusual findings promptly			

NOTES

PURPOSE

This chapter helps you learn the structure and function of the anus and rectum and the male prostate gland; the methods of inspection and palpation of these structures; and how to record the assessment accurately.

READING ASSIGNMENT

Jarvis: *Physical Examination and Health Assessment*, 6th ed., Chapter 25, pp. 709-724.

MEDIA ASSIGNMENT

Jarvis: *Physical Examination and Health Assessment* DVD Series: Male Genitalia.

GLOSSARY

Study the following terms after completing the reading assignment. You should be able to cover the definition on the right and define the term out loud.

Constipation . . . . decrease in stool frequency, with difficult passing of very hard, dry stools

Fissure . . . . painful longitudinal tear in tissue (e.g., in the superficial mucosa at the anal margin)

Hemorrhoid . . . . flabby papules of skin or mucous membrane in the anal region caused by a varicose vein of the hemorrhoidal plexus

Melena . . . . blood in the stool

Pruritus . . . . itching or burning sensation in the skin

Steatorrhea . . . . excessive fat in the stool as in gastrointestinal malabsorption of fat

Valves of Houston . . . . set of three semilunar transverse folds that cross one-half the circumference of the rectal lumen

STUDY GUIDE

After completing the reading assignment and the media assignment, you should be able to answer the following questions in the spaces provided.

1. State the length of the anal canal and the rectum in the adult, and describe the location of these structures in the lower abdomen.

2. Describe the size, shape, and location of the male prostate gland.

3. List a few examples of high-fiber foods of the soluble type and of the insoluble type; what advantages do these foods have for the body?

4. List screening measures that are recommended for early detection of colon/rectal cancer; of prostate cancer.

5. State the method of promoting anal sphincter relaxation to aid palpation of the anus and rectum.

Jarvis, Carolyn: PHYSICAL EXAMINATION AND HEALTH ASSESSMENT: Sixth Edition,
Student Laboratory Manual. Copyright © 2012, 2008, 2004, 2000, 1996 by Saunders, an imprint of Elsevier Inc. All rights reserved.

6. Describe the normal physical characteristics of the prostate gland that would be assessed by palpation:

Size

Shape

Surface

Consistency

Mobility

Sensitivity

7. Describe the physical appearance and clinical significance of pilonidal cyst and anorectal fistula.

8. Define the condition *benign prostatic hypertrophy,* list the usual symptoms the man experiences with this condition, and describe the physical characteristics.

Fill in the labels indicated on the following illustrations.

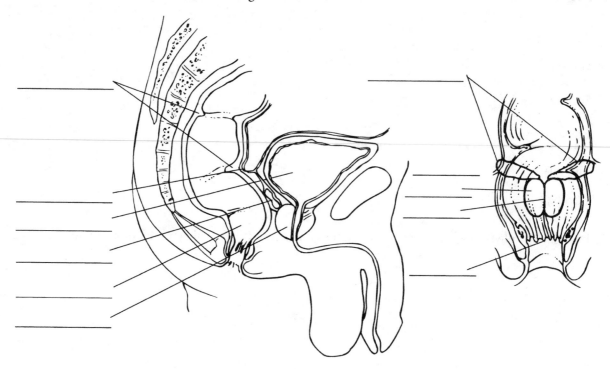

REVIEW QUESTIONS

This test is for you to check your own mastery of the content. Answers are provided in Appendix A.

1. The gastrocolic reflex is:

   a. a peristaltic wave.
   b. the passage of meconium in the newborn.
   c. another term for borborygmi.
   d. reverse peristalsis.

2. The incidence of benign prostatic hypertrophy (BPH) is highest among:

   a. European Americans.
   b. African Americans.
   c. Hispanics.
   d. Asians.

3. Select the best description of the anal canal.

   a. a 12-cm-long portion of the large intestine
   b. under involuntary control of the parasympathetic nervous system
   c. a 3.8-cm-long outlet of the gastrointestinal tract
   d. an S-shaped portion of the colon

4. While good nutrition is important for everyone, foods believed to help reduce risk of colon cancer are:

   a. high in fiber.
   b. low in fat.
   c. high in protein.
   d. high in carbohydrate.

5. Which finding in the prostate gland suggests prostate cancer?

   a. symmetric smooth enlargement
   b. extreme tenderness to palpation
   c. boggy soft enlargement
   d. diffuse hardness

6. The bulbourethral gland is assessed:

   a. during an examination of a female patient.
   b. during an examination of both male and female patients.
   c. during an examination of a male patient.
   d. cannot be assessed with a rectal examination.

7. Inspection of stool is an important part of the rectal examination. Normal stool is:

   a. black in color and tarry in consistency.
   b. brown in color and soft in consistency.
   c. clay colored and dry in consistency.
   d. varies depending upon the individual's diet.

8. Which symptoms suggest benign prostatic hypertrophy?

   a. weight loss and bone pain
   b. fever, chills, urinary frequency, and urgency
   c. difficulty initiating urination and weak stream
   d. dark, tarry stools

9. A false positive may occur on fecal occult blood tests of the stool if the person has ingested significant amounts of:

   a. red meat.
   b. candies with red dye #2.
   c. cranberry juice.
   d. red beets.

10. Write a narrative account of a rectal assessment with normal findings.

11. A patient states he is frequently constipated and when he has a bowel movement, he has rectal bleeding and pain. He does not feel any mass at his anal opening. "Do I have hemorrhoids, or is there something else wrong with me?" The examiner completes a rectal examination and explains that:

    a. there is an indication of rectal prolapse.
    b. it appears to be a pilonidal cyst.
    c. the symptoms are consistent with internal hemorrhoids.
    d. the problem is probably encopresis.

12. A patient states he has frothy, foul-smelling stools that float on the surface of the water in the toilet bowl. What condition is this patient describing?

    a. steatorrhea
    b. melena
    c. dyschezia
    d. a parasitic infection

SKILLS LABORATORY/CLINICAL SETTING

You are now ready for the clinical component of the rectal examination. This regional examination usually is combined with the examination of the male genitalia or with examination of the female genitalia.

Clinical Objectives

1. Demonstrate knowledge of the signs and symptoms related to the rectal area by obtaining a pertinent health history.

2. Inspect and palpate the perianal region.

3. Test any stool specimen for occult blood.

4. Record the history and physical examination findings accurately.

Instructions

Prepare the examination setting, and gather your equipment. Wash your hands; wear gloves during the examination; wash hands again after removing gloves. Practice the steps of the examination on a patient in the clinical setting, giving appropriate instructions as you proceed. Record your findings using the regional write-up sheet that follows. Note that only the worksheet is included in this chapter. Your narrative summary recording using the SOAP format can be included with the narrative summary of the genitalia.

NOTES

REGIONAL WRITE-UP—ANUS, RECTUM, AND PROSTATE GLAND

Date _____

Examiner _____

Patient _____ Age _____ Gender _____

Reason for visit _____

I. Health History

	No	Yes, explain
1. Bowels move **regularly**? How often?		
Usual color? Hard or soft?		
2. Any **change** in usual bowel habits?		
3. Ever had **black or bloody stool**?		
4. Take any medications?		
5. Any **rectal itching, pain, or hemorrhoids**?		
6. Any family history of **colon/rectal polyps or cancer**?		
7. Describe usual amount of high-fiber foods in diet.		

II. Physical Examination

A. Inspect the perianal area

Skin condition _____

Sacrococcygeal area _____

Note skin integrity while patient performs Valsalva maneuver _____

B. Palpate anus and rectum

Anal sphincter _____

Anal canal _____

Rectal wall _____

Prostate gland (for males)

    Size _____

    Shape _____

    Surface _____

    Consistency _____

    Mobility _____

    Any tenderness _____

Cervix (for females) _____

C. Examination of stool

Visual inspection _____

Test for occult blood _____

NOTES

PURPOSE

This chapter helps you learn the structure and function of the female genitalia; the methods of inspection and palpation of the internal and external structures; the procedures for collection of cytologic specimens; and how to record the assessment accurately.

READING ASSIGNMENT

Jarvis: *Physical Examination and Health Assessment*, 6th ed., Chapter 26, pp. 725-762.

MEDIA ASSIGNMENT

Jarvis: *Physical Examination and Health Assessment* DVD Series: Female Genitalia.

GLOSSARY

Study the following terms after completing the reading assignment. You should be able to cover the definition on the right and define the term out loud.

Adnexa . . . . accessory organs of the uterus (i.e., ovaries and fallopian tubes)

Amenorrhea . . . . absence of menstruation; termed *secondary amenorrhea* when menstruation has begun and then ceases; most common cause is pregnancy

Bartholin's glands . . . . vestibular glands, located on either side of the vaginal orifice, that secrete a clear lubricating mucus during intercourse

Bloody show . . . . dislodging of thick cervical mucus plug at end of pregnancy, which is a sign of beginning of labor

Caruncle . . . . small, deep red mass protruding from urethral meatus, usually due to urethritis

Chadwick sign . . . . bluish discoloration of cervix that occurs normally in pregnancy at 6 to 8 weeks' gestation

Chancre . . . . red, round, superficial ulcer with a yellowish serous discharge that is a sign of syphilis

Clitoris . . . . small, elongated erectile tissue in the female, located at anterior juncture of labia minora

Cystocele . . . . prolapse of urinary bladder and its vaginal mucosa into the vagina with straining or standing

Dysmenorrhea . . . . abdominal cramping and pain associated with menstruation

Dyspareunia . . . . painful intercourse

Dysuria . . . . painful urination

Endometriosis . . . . aberrant growths of endometrial tissue scattered throughout pelvis

Fibroid . . . . (myoma) hard, painless nodules in uterine wall that cause uterine enlargement

Gonorrhea . . . . sexually transmitted infection characterized by purulent vaginal discharge or may have no symptoms

Hegar sign . . . . softening of cervix that is a sign of pregnancy, occurring at 10 to 12 weeks' gestation

Hematuria . . . . red-tinged or bloody urine

Hymen . . . . membranous fold of tissue partly closing vaginal orifice

Leukorrhea . . . . whitish or yellowish discharge from vaginal orifice

Menarche . . . . onset of first menstruation, usually between 11 and 13 years of age

Menopause . . . . cessation of the menses, usually occurring around 48 to 51 years of age

Menorrhagia . . . . excessively heavy menstrual flow

Multipara . . . . condition of having two or more pregnancies

Nullipara . . . . condition of first pregnancy

Papanicolaou test . . . . painless test used to detect cervical cancer

Polyp . . . . cervical polyp is bright red, soft, pedunculated growth emerging from os

Rectocele . . . . prolapse of rectum and its vaginal mucosa into vagina with straining or standing

Rectouterine pouch . . . . (cul-de-sac of Douglas) deep recess formed by the peritoneum between the rectum and cervix

Salpingitis . . . . inflammation of fallopian tubes

Skene's glands . . . . paraurethral glands

Vaginitis . . . . inflammation of vagina

Vulva . . . . external genitalia of female

STUDY GUIDE

After completing the reading assignment and the media assignment, you should be able to answer the following questions in the spaces provided.

1. List and describe the external structures of the female genitalia.

2. Describe the size, shape, and location of the internal structures of the female genitalia.

3. Outline the changes observed during the perimenopausal period.

4. Discuss ways of creating an environment that will provide psychological comfort for both the woman and practitioner during the female genitalia examination.

5. Discuss selection, preparation, and insertion of the vaginal speculum.

6. Describe the appearance or *sketch* these normal variations of the cervix and os:

   Nulliparous _____

   Parous _____

   Stellate lacerations _____

   Cervical eversion _____

   Nabothian cysts _____

7. List the steps in the procedure of obtaining these specimens:

   Vaginal pool

   Cervical scrape using spatula

   Endocervical specimen using cytobrush

8. Contrast conventional glass-slide cytology with liquid-based cytology collection.

9. When applying acetic acid (white vinegar) to the cervix and vaginal mucosa, list the normal response and the response suggesting infection.

10. Discuss the procedure and rationale for bimanual examination and list normal findings for cervix, uterus, adnexa.

11. Discuss infection control precautions during examination of female genitalia and procuring of specimens.

12. Describe the appearance or *sketch* the appearance of the following abnormalities of the cervix:

Chadwick sign

Erosion

Polyp

Carcinoma

13. List the characteristics of vaginal discharge associated with the following conditions of vaginitis:

Candidiasis (yeast infection)

Trichomoniasis

Bacterial vaginosis

Chlamydia

Gonorrhea

14. Differentiate the signs and symptoms of these conditions of adnexal enlargement:

Ectopic pregnancy

Ovarian cyst

Fill in the labels indicated on the following illustrations.

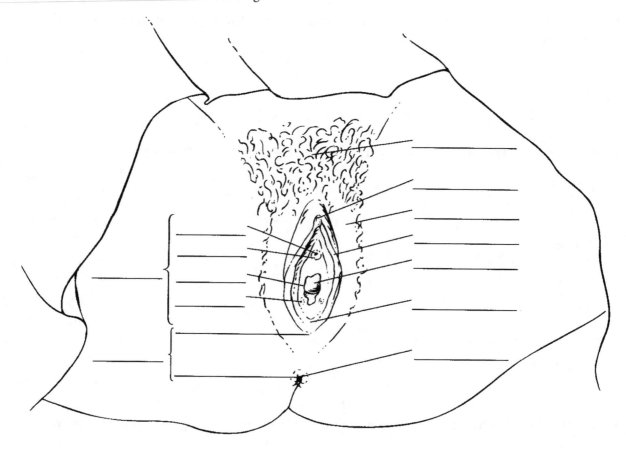

ANTERIOR VIEW OF ADNEXA

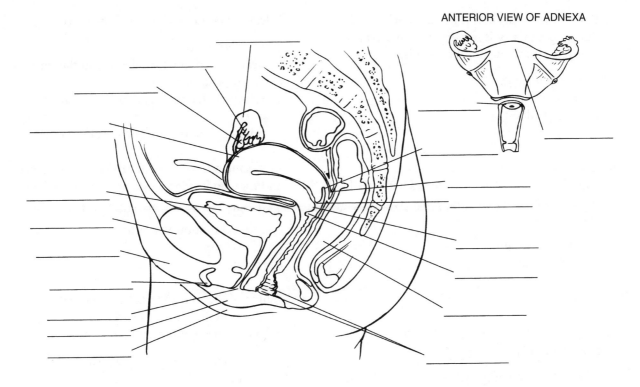

REVIEW QUESTIONS

This test is for you to check your own mastery of the content. Answers are provided in Appendix A.

1. Vaginal lubrication is provided during intercourse by:

    a. the labia minora.
    b. sebaceous follicles.
    c. Skene's glands.
    d. Bartholin's glands.

2. A young woman has come for her first gynecologic examination. Because she has not had any children, the examiner would expect the cervical os to appear:

    a. smooth and circular.
    b. irregular and slitlike.
    c. irregular and circular.
    d. smooth and enlarged.

3. A woman has come for an examination because of a missed menstrual period and a positive home pregnancy test. Examination reveals a cervix that appears cyanotic. This is referred to as:

    a. Goodell sign.
    b. Hegar sign.
    c. Tanner sign.
    d. Chadwick sign.

4. During the examination of the genitalia of a 70-year-old woman, a normal finding would be:

    a. hypertrophy of the mons pubis.
    b. increase in vaginal secretions.
    c. thin and sparse pubic hair.
    d. bladder prolapse.

5. For a woman, history of her mother's health during pregnancy is important. A medication that requires frequent follow-up is:

   a. corticosteroid.
   b. theophylline.
   c. diethylstilbestrol.
   d. aminoglycoside.

6. A woman has come for health care complaining of a thick, white discharge with intense itching. These symptoms are suggestive of:

   a. atrophic vaginitis.
   b. trichomoniasis.
   c. chlamydia.
   d. candidiasis.

7. To prepare the vaginal speculum for insertion, the examiner:

   a. lubricates it with a water-soluble lubricant.
   b. lubricates it with petrolatum.
   c. warms it under the light, then inserts it into the vagina.
   d. lubricates it with warm water.

8. To insert the speculum as comfortably as possible, the examiner:

   a. opens the speculum slightly and inserts in an upward direction.
   b. presses the introitus down with one hand and inserts the blades obliquely with the other.
   c. spreads the labia with one hand, inserts the closed speculum horizontally with the other.
   d. pushes down on the introitus and inserts the speculum in an upward direction.

9. Before withdrawing the speculum, the examiner swabs the cervix with a swab soaked in acetic acid. This examination is done to assess for:

   a. herpes simplex virus.
   b. contact dermatitis.
   c. human papillomavirus.
   d. carcinoma.

10. Select the best description of the uterus.

    a. anteverted, round asymmetric organ
    b. pear-shaped, thick-walled organ flattened anteroposteriorly
    c. retroverted, almond-shaped asymmetric organ
    d. midposition, thick-walled oval organ

11. In placing a finger on either side of the cervix and moving it side to side, you are assessing:

    a. the diameter of the fallopian tube.
    b. cervical motion tenderness.
    c. the ovaries.
    d. the uterus.

12. Which of the following is (are) normal, common finding(s) on inspection and palpation of the vulva and perineum?

    a. labia majora that are wide apart and gaping
    b. palpable Bartholin's glands
    c. clear, thin discharge from paraurethral glands
    d. bulging at introitus during Valsalva maneuver

13. Which of the following is the most common bacterial sexually transmitted infection in the United States?

    a. chlamydia
    b. gonorrhea
    c. trichomoniasis
    d. syphilis
    e. bacterial vaginosis

14. Write a narrative account of an assessment of female genitalia with normal findings.

15. What does the notation in a health record indicating the patient is a "G2 P3 Ab0" mean?

    a. The woman has delivered 3 children, 2 of whom are living; her blood type is Ab 0.
    b. The woman has been pregnant twice with 3 children (twins and another child), and all her children are living.
    c. The woman has been pregnant 3 times, has delivered 2 children, and had no abortions.
    d. The woman has been pregnant 3 times, has 2 living children, and had no spontaneous abortions.

16. What problems are associated with smoking and the use of oral contraceptives?

    a. increased risk of alcoholism and cirrhosis of the liver
    b. thrombophlebitis and pulmonary emboli
    c. infertility and weight gain
    d. urinary tract infections and skin cancer

SKILLS LABORATORY/CLINICAL SETTING

You are now ready for the clinical component of the female genitalia examination. Because of the need to maintain personal privacy, it is likely you will not practice this examination on a peer. Your practice likely will be with a teaching mannequin in the skills laboratory or with a woman in the clinical setting under the guidance of a preceptor. Before you proceed, discuss the feelings that may be experienced by the woman and examiner and methods to increase the comfort of both. With your instructor, discuss methods of positioning the woman, steps in using the vaginal speculum, steps in procuring specimens, and methods of infection control precautions.

Clinical Objectives

1. Demonstrate knowledge of the signs and symptoms related to the female genitalia by obtaining a pertinent health history.

2. Demonstrate measures to increase the woman's comfort before and during the examination.

3. Demonstrate knowledge of infection control precautions before, during, and after the examination.

4. Inspect and palpate the external genitalia.

5. Using the vaginal speculum, gather materials for cytologic study.

6. Inspect and palpate the internal genitalia.

7. Record the history and physical examination findings accurately, reach an assessment of the health state, and develop a plan of care.

Instructions

Prepare the examination setting, and gather your equipment. Collect the health history before the woman disrobes for the examination. Wash your hands; wear gloves during the examination; wash hands again after removing gloves. Practice the steps of the examination on a woman in the clinical setting, giving appropriate instructions as you proceed. Record your findings using the regional write-up sheet that follows. The first section is intended as a worksheet; the last page is intended for your narrative summary recording using the SOAP format. Collection of data for the rectal examination is usually combined with the examination of female genitalia; see Chapter 25 for the regional write-up sheet for the rectal examination.

NOTES

REGIONAL WRITE-UP—FEMALE GENITOURINARY SYSTEM

Date _____

Examiner _____

Patient _____ Age _____ Gender _____

Reason for visit _____

I. Health History

	No	Yes, explain
1. Date of **last menstrual period?**		
Age at first period? Usual cycle?		
Duration? Usual amount of flow?		
Any pain or cramps with period?		
2. Ever been **pregnant**? How many times?		
Describe pregnancy(ies)		
Any complications?		
3. Periods slowed down or **stopped**?		
4. How often has **gynecologic checkup**?		
Date of last Pap test? Results?		
5. Any problems with **urinating**?		
6. Any unusual **vaginal discharge**?		
7. **Sores or lesions** in genitals?		
8. In relationship now involving intercourse?		
9. Use a contraceptive? Which one?		
10. Any contact with partner who has sexually transmitted infection?		
11. Any precautions to reduce risk of STIs?		
12. Taking any medications?		
Any hormone therapy?		

II. Physical Examination
A. Inspect external genitalia
Skin color and characteristics _____
Hair distribution _____
Symmetry _____
Clitoris _____
Labia _____
Urethral opening _____
Vaginal opening _____
Perineum _____

B. Palpate external genitalia
Skene's glands _____
Bartholin's glands _____
Perineum _____
Assess perineal muscle strength _____
Assess for vaginal wall bulging or urinary incontinence _____
Discharge and characteristics _____

C. Speculum examination
Inspect cervix and os
    Color _____
    Position _____
    Size _____
    Surface _____
    Discharge and characteristics _____
Obtain cervical smears and cultures
    Vaginal pool _____
    Cervical scrape _____
    Endocervical specimen _____
    Other (if indicated) _____
Complete acetic acid wash _____
Inspect vaginal wall as speculum is removed _____

D. Bimanual examination
Cervix
    Consistency _____
    Mobility _____
    Tenderness with motion _____
Uterus
    Size and shape _____
    Consistency _____
    Position _____
    Mobility _____
    Tenderness _____
Adnexa
    Able to palpate? (Be honest.) _____
    Size and shape of ovaries _____
    Tenderness _____
    Masses _____
Rectovaginal examination _____

REGIONAL WRITE-UP—FEMALE GENITOURINARY SYSTEM

Summarize your findings using the SOAP format.

Subjective (Reason for seeking care, health history)

Objective (Physical examination findings)   Record findings on diagram below

Assessment (Assessment of health state or problem, diagnosis)

Plan (Diagnostic evaluation, follow-up care, patient teaching)

NOTES

CHAPTER

27

The Complete Health Assessment: Putting It All Together

PURPOSE

This chapter helps you learn the methods of integrating the regional examinations so that you will be able to conduct a complete physical examination on a well young adult.

READING ASSIGNMENT

Jarvis: *Physical Examination and Health Assessment*, 6th ed., Chapter 27, pp. 763-786.

MEDIA ASSIGNMENT

Jarvis: *Physical Examination and Health Assessment* DVD Series: Head-to-Toe Examination of the Adult.

CLINICAL OBJECTIVES

1. Demonstrate skills of inspection, percussion, palpation, and auscultation.

2. Demonstrate correct use of instruments, including assembly, manipulation of component parts, and positioning with patient.

3. Use appropriate terminology and correctly pronounce medical terminology with clinical instructor and with patient.

4. Choreograph the complete examination in a systematic manner, including integration of certain regional assessments throughout the examination (e.g., skin, musculoskeletal).

5. Coordinate procedures to limit position changes for examiner and patient.

6. Describe accurately the findings of the examination, including normal and abnormal findings.

7. Demonstrate appropriate infection control measures.

8. Recognize and maintain the privacy and dignity of the patient.

   a. Adequately explain what is being done while limiting small talk.
   b. Consider patient's anxiety and fears.
   c. Consider your own facial expression and comments.
   d. Demonstrate confidence, empathy, and gentle manner.
   e. Acknowledge and apologize for any discomfort caused.
   f. Provide for privacy and warmth at all times.
   g. Determine comfort level, pausing if patient becomes tired.
   h. Wash hands and don gloves appropriately.
   i. Allow adequate time for each step.
   j. Briefly summarize findings to patient, and thank patient for his or her time.

INSTRUCTIONS

The key to success in this venture is **practice;** you should conduct at least **three** complete physical examination practices in your preparation for this final examination proficiency. You are responsible for obtaining a peer "patient" for the examination. You should prepare your own note card "outline" for the examination. You may refer to this minimally during the examination, but overdependence on your notes will constitute failure. You will have 45 minutes in which to conduct the examination (not including setup). Genitalia examination is omitted. If you practice three times, you will have no difficulty completing the examination in the allotted time.

Prepare the examination setting. Arrange for proper lighting. If you are using a hospital bed instead of an examination table, make sure to adjust the bed height during the examination to allow for your own visualization of the patient and for the patient's ease in getting into and out of the bed. Arrange adequate patient gown, bath blankets, and drapes.

Gather your equipment. The following items are needed for a complete physical examination, including female genitalia. Check with your clinical instructor for any items that you may omit for your own examination proficiency.

Platform scale with height attachment	Skin-marking pen
Sphygmomanometer with appropriate-size cuff	Flexible tape measure and ruler marked in centimeters
Stethoscope with bell and diaphragm endpieces	Reflex hammer
Alcohol wipes for cleaning equipment	Sharp object (split tongue blade)
Thermometer	Cotton balls
Flashlight or penlight	Bivalve vaginal speculum
Otoscope/ophthalmoscope	Disposable gloves
Tuning fork	Materials for cytologic study
Nasal speculum	Lubricant
Tongue depressor	Fecal occult blood test materials
Pocket vision screener	

Record your findings using the write-up sheets that follow. Your clinical instructor may ask you to record your findings ahead of time, following one of your practice sessions. Then you can give your write-up to the instructor to follow along as you perform the final examination proficiency.

Good luck!

COMPLETE PHYSICAL EXAMINATION

Date _____

Examiner _____

Patient _____ Age _____ Gender _____

Occupation _____ Reason for visit _____

General Survey of Patient

1. Appears stated age _____
2. Level of consciousness _____
3. Skin color _____
4. Nutritional status _____
5. Posture and position _____
6. Obvious physical deformities _____
7. Mobility: gait, use of assistive devices, ROM of joints, no involuntary movement _____
8. Facial expression _____
9. Mood and affect _____
10. Speech: articulation, pattern, content appropriate, native language _____
11. Hearing _____
12. Personal hygiene _____

Measurement and Vital Signs

1. Weight _____
2. Height _____
3. Waist circumference _____
4. Body mass index _____
5. Vision using Snellen eye chart _____
   Right eye _____ Left eye _____ Correction? _____
6. Radial pulse, rate, and rhythm _____
7. Respirations, rate, depth _____
8. Blood pressure
   Right arm _____ (sitting or lying?)
   Left arm _____ (sitting or lying?)
9. Temperature (if indicated) _____
10. Pain assessment _____

Stand in Front of Patient, Patient Is Sitting

Skin

1. Hands and nails _____
2. (For remainder of examination, examine skin with corresponding region)
   Color and pigmentation _____
   Temperature _____
   Moisture _____
   Texture _____
   Turgor _____
   Any lesions _____

Head and Face
1. Scalp, hair, cranium _____
2. Face (cranial nerve VII) _____
3. Temporal artery, temporomandibular joint _____
4. Maxillary sinuses, frontal sinuses _____

Eyes
1. Visual fields (cranial nerve II) _____
2. Extraocular muscles, corneal light reflex _____
   Cardinal positions of gaze (cranial nerves III, IV, VI) _____
3. External structures _____
4. Conjunctivae _____
   Sclerae _____
   Corneas _____
   Irides _____
5. Pupils _____
6. Ophthalmoscope, red reflex _____
   Disc _____
   Vessels _____
   Retinal background _____

Ears
1. External ear _____
2. Any tenderness _____
3. Otoscope, ear canal _____
   Tympanic membrane _____
4. Test hearing (cranial nerve VIII), voice test _____

Nose
1. External nose _____
2. Patency of nostrils _____
3. Speculum, nasal mucosa _____
   Septum _____
   Turbinates _____

Mouth and Throat
1. Lips and buccal mucosa _____
   Teeth and gums _____
   Tongue _____
   Hard/soft palate _____
2. Tonsils _____
3. Uvula (cranial nerves IX, X) _____
4. Tongue (cranial nerve XII) _____

Neck
1. Symmetry, lumps, pulsations _____
2. Cervical lymph nodes _____
3. Carotid pulse (bruits if indicated) _____
4. Trachea _____
5. ROM and muscle strength (cranial nerve XI) _____

Move to Back of Patient, Patient Sitting

6. Thyroid gland _____

Chest and Lungs, Posterior and Lateral

1. Thoracic cage configuration _____
   Skin characteristics _____
   Symmetry _____
2. Symmetric expansion _____
   Tactile fremitus _____
   Lumps or tenderness _____
3. Spinous processes _____
4. Percussion over lung fields _____
   Diaphragmatic excursion _____
5. CVA tenderness _____
6. Breath sounds _____
7. Adventitious sounds _____

Move to Front of Patient

Chest and Lungs, Anterior

1. Respirations and skin characteristics _____
2. Tactile fremitus, lumps, tenderness _____
3. Percuss lung fields _____
4. Breath sounds _____

Upper Extremities

1. ROM and muscle strength _____
2. Epitrochlear nodes _____

Breasts

1. Symmetry, mobility, dimpling _____
2. Supraclavicular and infraclavicular areas _____

Patient Supine, Stand at Patient's Right

3. Breast palpation _____
4. Nipple _____
5. Axillae and regional nodes _____
6. Teach breast self-examination _____

Neck Vessels

1. Jugular venous pulse _____
2. Jugular venous pressure, if indicated _____

Heart

1. Precordium: pulsations and heave _____
2. Apical impulse _____
3. Precordium, thrills _____

   4. Apical rate and rhythm _____
   5. Heart sounds _____

Abdomen
   1. Contour, symmetry _____
      Skin characteristics _____
      Umbilicus and pulsations _____
   2. Bowel sounds _____
   3. Vascular sounds _____
   4. Percussion _____
   5. Liver span in right MCL _____
   6. Spleen _____
   7. Light and deep palpation _____
   8. Palpation of liver, spleen, kidneys, aorta _____
   9. Abdominal reflexes, if indicated _____

Inguinal Area
   1. Femoral pulse _____
   2. Inguinal nodes _____

Lower Extremities
   1. Symmetry _____
      Skin characteristics, hair distribution _____
   2. Pulses, popliteal _____
      Posterior tibial _____
      Dorsalis pedis _____
   3. Temperature, pretibial edema _____
   4. Toes _____

Patient Sits Up

   5. ROM and muscle strength, hips _____
      Knees _____
      Ankles and feet _____

Neurologic
   1. Sensation, face _____
      Arms and hands _____
      Legs and feet _____
   2. Position sense _____
   3. Stereognosis _____
   4. Cerebellar function, finger-to-nose _____
   5. Cerebellar function, heel-to-shin _____
   6. Deep tendon reflexes
      Biceps _____   Triceps _____
      Brachioradialis _____   Patellar _____
      Achilles _____
   7. Babinski reflex _____

Patient Stands Up

Musculoskeletal

1. Walk across room _____
   Walk, heel to toe _____
2. Walk on tiptoes, and then walk on heels _____
3. Romberg sign _____
4. Shallow knee bend _____
5. Touch toes _____
6. ROM of spine _____

Male Genitalia

1. Penis and scrotum _____
2. Testes and spermatic cord _____
3. Inguinal hernia _____
4. Teach testicular self-examination _____

Male Rectum

1. Perianal area _____
2. Rectal walls and prostate gland _____
3. Stool for occult blood _____

Female Patient in Lithotomy Position

Female Genitalia and Rectum

1. Perineal and perianal areas _____
2. Vaginal speculum: cervix and vaginal walls _____
3. Procure specimens _____
4. Bimanual: cervix, uterus, and adnexa _____
   _____
5. Rectovaginal _____
6. Stool for occult blood _____

Closure

1. Help patient sit up
2. Thank patient for time, and depart from patient

NOTES

CHAPTER 28

Bedside Assessment of the Hospitalized Adult

PURPOSE

This chapter helps you learn the methods of integrating the regional examinations in the manner that suits the inpatient setting. The selection and sequencing of the techniques included are structured to provide an assessment that is efficient, thorough, and consistent with the assessments performed by other nurses in the course of 24-hour care.

READING ASSIGNMENT

Jarvis: *Physical Examination and Health Assessment*, 6th ed., Chapter 28, pp. 787-794.

CLINICAL OBJECTIVES

1. Demonstrate skills of inspection, percussion, palpation, and auscultation.

2. Demonstrate correct use of instruments, including assembly, manipulation of component parts, and positioning with patient.

3. Use appropriate terminology and correctly pronounce medical terminology with clinical instructor and with patient.

4. Choreograph the complete examination in a systematic manner, including integration of certain regional assessments throughout the examination (e.g., skin, musculoskeletal).

5. Coordinate procedures to limit position changes for examiner and patient.

6. Describe accurately the findings of the examination, including normal and abnormal findings.

7. Demonstrate appropriate infection control measures.

8. Recognize and maintain the privacy and dignity of the patient.

   a. Adequately explain what is being done while limiting small talk.
   b. Consider patient's anxiety and fears.
   c. Consider your own facial expression and comments.
   d. Demonstrate confidence, empathy, and gentle manner.

   e. Acknowledge and apologize for any discomfort caused.

   f. Provide for privacy and warmth at all times.

   g. Determine comfort level, pausing if patient becomes tired.

   h. Wash hands and don gloves appropriately.

   i. Allow adequate time for each step.

   j. Briefly summarize findings to patient, and thank patient for his or her time.

9. Complete all procedures with attention to specifics of technique, which allows clear and consistent replication of the procedures by others assessing the same patient.

INSTRUCTIONS

As with other assessments, this particular version of the head-to-toe examination requires a great deal of practice before you will feel truly confident. The good news about this sequence is that it is directly applicable in any inpatient clinical sites that you attend, which is likely to be most of them. If you are already attending clinicals, use any available time to practice this sequence on real patients.

You are responsible for recruiting a friend or classmate to act as your patient for this examination. Prepare an outline on a note card to help you remember the sequence. Do not use it as a step-by-step instruction but, rather, as a double-check so that you do not omit anything. Once this examination is over, you can take the note card with you to clinicals and use it as a reference.

You will have 20 minutes for this examination, not including setup. If you have practiced the individual regional assessments thoroughly and can complete this particular sequence three times, you will be able to complete it satisfactorily within the time allotted.

Prepare the examination setting. Arrange the lighting, furniture, and bed to allow for the most efficient and comfortable activity for yourself and your patient. Think carefully about the functions of the patient's hospital bed. It can be useful to raise the bed closer to your eyes and stethoscope, but you cannot expect the patient to get out of bed safely from that height. Position sheets, drapes, and bath blankets strategically to achieve the proper balance of modesty, efficiency, and comfort.

Gather and arrange your equipment before you begin. The following items are needed for this sequence, but your instructor may modify the equipment list slightly for your individual class or exercise.

Water (in a cup)	Ruler in millimeters
Watch with a second hand	Oxygen equipment (as indicated by your instructor)
Stethoscope	Doppler (as indicated by your instructor)
Blood pressure cuff	Bladder scanner (as indicated by your instructor)
Pulse oximeter	Standardized scales to calculate patient's risk for skin breakdown and falling
Penlight	Documentation forms (as included here, or provided by your instructor)

Verify with your instructor whether you should submit documentation of this particular assessment after your demonstration or documentation that you have prepared to reflect one of your earlier practice sessions.

Good luck!

COMPLETE INPATIENT REASSESSMENT

Date _____

Examiner _____

Patient _____ Age _____ Gender _____

Occupation _____ Reason for admission _____

Introduction
1. Check for flags or markers at doorway
2. Introduce yourself
3. Perform hand hygiene
4. Make eye contact
5. Offer water
6. Check name band
7. Ask appropriate interview questions, including current pain
8. Elevate the bed to appropriate height

General Appearance
1. Facial expression _____
2. Body position _____
3. Level of consciousness _____
4. Skin color _____
5. Nutritional status _____
6. Speech: articulation, pattern, content appropriate _____
7. Hearing _____
8. Personal hygiene _____

Measurement
1. Temperature _____
2. Pulse _____
3. Respiration _____
4. Blood pressure _____
5. Pulse oximetry _____
6. Weight on admission or if daily weight is indicated _____
7. Rate pain level on 1-to-10 scale; note ability to tolerate pain _____
8. Pain reassessment, if appropriate to scenario _____

Neurologic System
1. Eyes open:
   a. Spontaneously _____
   b. Name _____
2. Motor response _____
3. Verbal response _____
4. Pupil size in mm and reaction
   a. R _____ b. L _____
5. Upper muscle strength
   a. R _____ b. L _____

6. Lower muscle strength
   a. R _____   b. L _____
7. Any ptosis, facial droop _____
8. Sensation _____
9. Communication _____
10. Ability to swallow _____

Respiratory

1. Oxygen by mask, nasal prongs; check fitting _____
2. FIo_2 _____
3. Respiratory effort _____
4. Auscultate breath sounds:
   Anterior lobes:
      Right upper _____
      Left upper _____
      Right middle _____
      Right lower _____
      Left lower _____
   Posterior lobes:
      Left upper _____
      Right upper _____
      Left lower _____
      Right lower _____
   Cough and deep breathe; any mucus? Check color and amount _____
   Educate on use of incentive spirometry if ordered

Cardiovascular System

1. Auscultate rhythm at apex: regular, irregular? _____
2. Check apical versus radial pulse
3. Assess heart sounds in all auscultatory areas: first with diaphragm, repeat with bell
4. Check capillary refill _____
5. Check pretibial edema
   a. R _____   b. L _____
6. Palpate posterior tibial pulse
   a. R _____   b. L _____
7. Palpate dorsalis pedis pulse
   a. R _____   b. L _____
8. Pulses by Doppler, if assigned _____
9. IV fluid and rate, if present _____

Skin (may be integrated with rest of assessment)

1. Color _____
2. Temperature _____
3. Pinch up a fold of skin under the clavicle or on the forearm _____
4. Note any lesions; check any dressings _____
5. Note skin around IV site _____
6. Standardized scale regarding skin breakdown _____
7. Settings and application of specialized surface, if present _____

Abdomen

1. Contour of abdomen: flat, rounded, protuberant _____
2. Bowel sounds in all four quadrants _____
3. Check any tube drainage and site _____
4. Inquire if passing flatus or stool _____
5. Can patient tolerate current diet? Should diet be advanced or changed? _____

Genitourinary

1. Inquire if voiding regularly _____
2. Urine for color, clarity, quantity _____
3. Bladder scan, if indicated _____

Activity

1. If on bedrest, check head of bed, risk for skin breakdown _____
2. Any SCDs, TED hose, foot pumps? Must be hooked up/on _____
3. Transfer to chair _____
4. Note any assistance needed, how movement is tolerated, distance walked to chair, ability to turn _____
5. Need for any ambulatory aid or equipment _____
6. Standardized scale regarding falling _____

Closure

1. Return bed to lowest height
2. Verify that brakes are locked
3. Make sure appropriate rails are up
4. Ensure call bell is available
5. Verify bed alarm, if indicated
6. Thank the patient for his/her attention and cooperation
7. Initiate or continue appropriate Plan of Care
8. Complete assessment and document into computer

NOTES

PURPOSE

This chapter helps you learn the changes and function of the female genitalia during pregnancy; the methods of inspection and palpation of the internal and external structures and the maternal abdomen; and how to record the assessment accurately.

READING ASSIGNMENT

Jarvis: *Physical Examination and Health Assessment,* 6th ed., Chapter 29, pp. 795-828.

MEDIA ASSIGNMENT

Jarvis: *Physical Examination and Health Assessment* DVD Series: Head-to-Toe Examination of the Pregnant Woman.

GLOSSARY

Study the following terms after completing the reading assignment. You should be able to cover the definition on the right and define the term out loud.

Amniocentesis. . . . . the transabdominal perforation of the amniotic sac for the purpose of obtaining a sample of amniotic fluid

Antenatal testing . . . . consists of monitoring fetal growth, amniotic fluid volume, umbilical cord Doppler blood flow, and fetal monitoring via non-stress or contraction stress testing using a fetal monitor

Antepartum. . . . . the period occurring before childbirth

Blastocyst. . . . . the fertilized ovum; a specialized layer of cells around the blastocyst becomes the placenta

Cervical biopsy. . . . . removal of a small piece of tissue from the cervix to analyze for abnormal cells

Cervical cerclage. . . . . a strong stitch inserted into and around the cervix in early pregnancy for the treatment of cervical insufficiency

Chadwick sign . . . . bluish purple discoloration of the cervix during pregnancy due to venous congestion

Chloasma. . . . . the "mask of pregnancy"; butterfly-shaped pigmentation of the face

Chorionic villi sampling. . . . . . transabdominal or transvaginal sampling of trophoblastic tissue surrounding the gestational sac

Colostrum. . . . . the precursor to milk that contains minerals, proteins, and antibodies

Corpus luteum . . . . "yellow body"; a structure on the surface of the ovary that is formed by the remaining cells in the follicle; it acts as a short-lived endocrine organ that produces progesterone to help maintain the pregnancy in its early stages

Diastasis recti . . . . separation of the abdominal muscles during pregnancy, returning to normal after pregnancy

Engagement. . . . . when the widest diameter of the presenting part has descended into the pelvic inlet

Fetal lie. . . . . orientation of the fetal spine to the maternal spine

Goodell sign . . . . the softening of the cervix due to increased vascularity, congestion, and edema

Hegar sign . . . . when the uterus becomes globular in shape, softens, and flexes easily over the cervix

Hyperemesis gravidarum . . . . . severe and debilitating nausea and vomiting that may persist beyond the 14th week of pregnancy and cause dehydration, weight loss, and electrolyte imbalance

Intrapartum . . . . occurring during labor and delivery

LEEP procedure . . . . loop electrical excision procedure; uses a thin, low-voltage electrified wire loop to cut out abnormal tissue of the cervix; not done during pregnancy

Leopold maneuver . . . . external palpation of the maternal abdomen to determine fetal lie, presentation, attitude, and position

Linea nigra . . . . a median line of the abdomen that becomes pigmented (darkens) during pregnancy

"Morning sickness" . . . . nausea and vomiting of pregnancy that usually begins between weeks 4 and 6, peaks between weeks 8 and 12, and resolves between weeks 14 and 16

Mucus plug . . . . mucus that forms a thick barrier in the cervix that is expelled at various times before or during labor

Multigravida. . . . . a pregnant woman who has previously carried a fetus to the point of viability

Multipara. . . . . a woman who has had two or more viable pregnancies and deliveries

Nägele's rule . . . . a rule for calculating the estimated date of delivery; add 7 days to the first day of the last menstrual period and subtract 3 months

Nuchal translucency. . . . . the amount of fluid behind the neck of the fetus; also known as the *nuchal fold*. Fetuses at risk for Down syndrome tend to have a higher amount of fluid

Pelvimetry. . . . . assessment of the maternal pelvis bones for shape and size

Pica. . . . . a craving for unnatural articles of food, such as cornstarch and ice chips

Position . . . . the location of a fetal part to the right or left of the maternal pelvis

Postpartum . . . . the period occurring after delivery

Presentation . . . . the part of the fetus that is entering the pelvis first

Primigravida . . . . a woman pregnant for the first time

Primipara . . . . a woman who has had one pregnancy and delivery

Sequential screening . . . . a method of prenatal risk screening using maternal serum and ultrasound

Striae gravidarum . . . . "stretch marks" that may be seen on the abdomen and breasts (in areas of weight gain) during pregnancy

VBAC . . . . vaginal birth after cesarean delivery

STUDY GUIDE

After completing the reading assignment and the media assignment, you should be able to answer the following questions in the spaces provided.

1. Describe the function of the placenta.

2. Using Nägele's rule, calculate the estimated date of delivery if the LMP is August 22.

3. Give examples of the following signs of pregnancy.

   Presumptive: _____

   Probable: _____

   Positive: _____

4. When can serum hCG be detected in maternal blood?

5. Describe three physical and physiologic changes that are seen in the:

   First trimester: _____

   Second trimester: _____

   Third trimester: _____

6. Describe the "recommended" weight gain during pregnancy.

7. List the major concerns for teenage maternal morbidity and mortality.

8. List at least 3 risk factors concerning pregnant women of advanced maternal age.

9. Discuss the importance of how transcultural differences play a role in a woman's pregnancy.

10. List at least 3 ways in which you as a health care provider can be culturally sensitive to a woman during her antepartum, intrapartum, and postpartum periods.

11. True or False: Please circle the best answer.

    True   False   A woman who has had a classic uterine incision is a good candidate for a VBAC.

    True   False   In early fetal development, the corpus luteum plays no significance.

    True   False   A woman who is pregnant for the first time is called a *primipara*.

    True   False   The fetal period begins after the 9th gestational week.

    True   False   Preeclampsia is seen only in the third trimester of pregnancy.

    True   False   Vaginal bleeding in pregnancy always indicates a miscarriage.

    True   False   Cervical incompetence is always accompanied by painful contractions.

12. What is the importance of fetal movement counting, and when should it be initiated?

13. Describe why it is important to ask a pregnant woman if she feels safe in her relationships and environment.

14. Draw on this diagram where the fundal height should be at the 20th week of gestation.

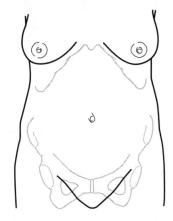

15. Label the following types of pelvis.

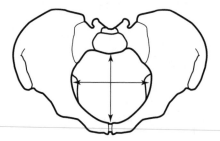   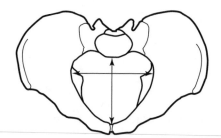

_____   _____

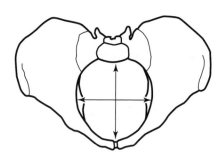   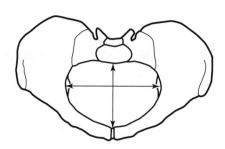

_____   _____

16. Label, list the order, and describe the purpose of the following maneuvers.

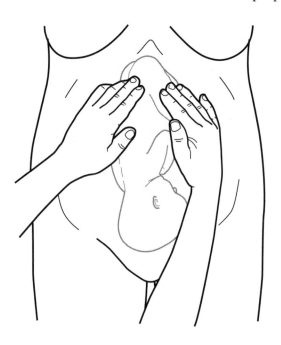   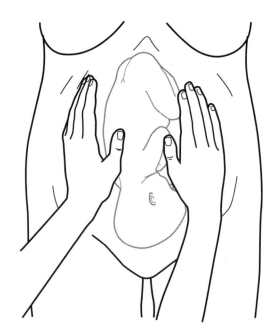

_____   _____

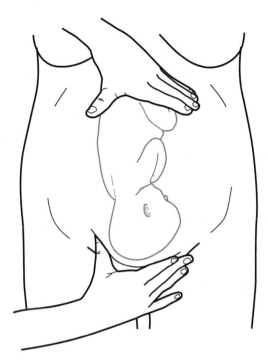

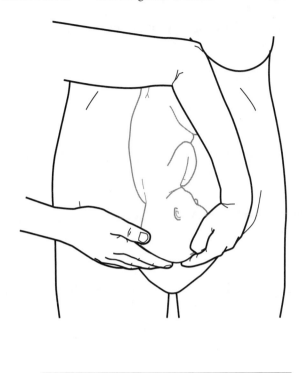

_____

_____

17. Describe the following for this figure.

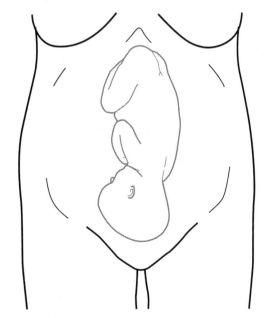

Fetal lie: _____

Fetal presentation: _____

Fetal position: _____

18. List the symptoms of preeclampsia.

19. List at least 2 reasons why fundal height may be small for gestational age.

20. List at least 2 reasons why fundal height may be large for gestational age.

REVIEW QUESTIONS

This test is for you to check your own mastery of the content. Answers are provided in Appendix A.

1. Ovulation begins on the:

   a. 1st day of the menstrual cycle.
   b. 28th day of the menstrual cycle.
   c. 14th day/approximately of the menstrual cycle.

2. Using Nägele's rule, the estimated date of delivery (EDD) if a woman's last menstrual period started on January 13 is:

   a. $1/13 + 7 = 20$ $20 - 3$ months   EDD = October ≈ 29
   b. $1/13 + 10 = 23$ $23 - 3$ months   EDD = October ≈ 18
   c. $1/13 + 14 = 27$ $27 - 3$ months   EDD = September ≈ 30

3. A woman comes to the clinic complaining of nausea, fatigue, breast tenderness, urinary frequency, and amenorrhea. These are:

   a. probable signs of pregnancy.
   b. positive signs of pregnancy.
   c. presumptive signs of pregnancy.
   d. signs of stress.

4. After implantation, what structure makes progesterone to support the pregnancy up until week 10?

   a. corpus luteum
   b. blastocyst
   c. placenta
   d. ovary

5. Approximately 2 to 3 weeks before labor, the woman will experience:

   a. extreme fatigue.
   b. Braxton-Hicks contractions.
   c. lightening.
   d. back pain.

6. Cardiac output in a pregnant woman:

   a. drops dramatically.
   b. remains the same.
   c. increases along with stroke volume.
   d. decreases along with stroke volume.
   e. none of the above.

7. The pregnant adolescent is medically at risk for:

   a. poor weight gain, preeclampsia, thyroiditis, miscarriage.
   b. poor weight gain, preeclampsia, sexually transmitted infections.
   c. stress, abuse, inadequate housing, inadequate education.
   d. miscarriage, hypothyroidism, poor weight gain.

8. Women older than 35 years who desire a pregnancy are at increased risk for:

   a. congenital anomalies.
   b. infertility.
   c. diabetes.
   d. hypertension.
   e. all of the above.

9. Sexually transmitted infections place the pregnant woman at risk for:

   a. infertility.
   b. premature rupture of membranes.
   c. preterm labor.
   d. preterm delivery.
   e. all of the above.
   f. b, c, and d.

10. Abdominal pain in the first trimester may be indicative of:

    a. preterm labor.
    b. ectopic pregnancy.
    c. appendicitis.
    d. urinary tract infection.
    e. all of the above.
    f. b, c, and d.

11. A woman at approximately 20 weeks' gestation who is complaining of lower right and/or left quadrant pain may be experiencing:

    a. appendicitis.
    b. constipation.
    c. urinary tract infection.
    d. stretching of the round ligament.
    e. none of the above.

12. You are palpating the maternal abdomen at approximately 35 weeks. Your left hand is on the maternal right, and your right hand is on the maternal left. What maneuver is this?

    a. Leopold's first maneuver
    b. Leopold's second maneuver
    c. Schmidt's third maneuver
    d. Schmidt's second maneuver

13. Fetal heart tones are best auscultated over the fetal:

    a. back.
    b. abdomen.
    c. shoulder.

14. Chadwick sign is:

    a. softening of the cervix.
    b. rotation of the cervix to the left.
    c. fundus of the uterus tips forward.
    d. a bluish color of the cervix and vaginal walls during early pregnancy.

15. An obstetric ultrasound is done to determine:

    a. thickness of the uterine wall.
    b. fetal position.
    c. placental location.
    d. amniotic fluid volume.
    e. none of the above.
    f. b, c, and d.

16. Write a narrative account of some abnormal findings in pregnancy. List possible causes and consequences to the mother and fetus.

SKILLS LABORATORY/CLINICAL SETTING

You are now ready for the clinical component of the pregnant female examination. Because of the need to maintain personal privacy, it is unlikely you will practice this examination on a peer. Some clinical settings may arrange for pregnant women to participate, or your practice setting may have available a pregnant teaching mannequin that you may use to practice your skills. If you have a pregnant woman available, discuss with her, in the presence of your instructor, the methods of examination that will be used. Maintain her comfort and adequate positioning to prevent maternal dizziness, nausea, and hypotension and to maintain adequate uterine blood flow.

Clinical Objectives

1. Demonstrate the knowledge of the physical changes related to pregnancy in the first, second, and third trimesters.

2. Demonstrate the knowledge and importance of obtaining a pertinent health history during the first prenatal visit.

3. Demonstrate cultural sensitivity during the examination.

4. Inspect and palpate the maternal abdomen for uterine size and fetal position.

5. Demonstrate obtaining fetal heart tones.

6. Record the history and physical examination findings accurately; reach an assessment of the health state, estimated gestational age, and fetal position (when appropriate); and develop a plan of care.

Instructions

Prepare the examination setting, and gather your equipment. Collect the health history before the woman disrobes for the examination. Calculate the EDD. Wash your hands. Practice the steps of the examination on a woman in the clinical setting, giving appropriate instructions and explanations as you proceed. Record your findings using the regional write-up sheet that follows. The first section is intended as a worksheet; the last page is intended for your narrative summary recording using the SOAP format. See Chapter 26 for the female genital examination.

REGIONAL WRITE-UP—PREGNANT FEMALE

_____

Patient Name   Date

PRENATAL HISTORY QUESTIONNAIRE

Having a healthy baby is a special event. Once a baby is born, families take certain precautions to ensure the baby's health and safety. The unborn child deserves similar care.

QUESTIONNAIRE

The following questions will help in the care of your pregnancy. Please answer these questions as well as you can. All answers will remain private. If you need help answering the questions, please ask your health care provider. The first question relates to your family history. The next 7 questions will be about you, your baby's father, and both your families. When thinking about your families, please include your child (or unborn baby), mother, father, sisters, brothers, grandparents, aunts, uncles, nieces, nephews, and cousins.

Yes   No   1.   Will you be 35 years or older when the baby is due? Age when due: _____ .

Yes   No   2.   Are you and the baby's father related to each other (e.g., cousins)?

Yes   No   3.   Have you had three or more pregnancies that ended in miscarriage?

Yes   No   4.   Have you or the baby's father had a stillborn baby or a baby who died around the time of delivery?

Yes   No   5.   Do either you or the baby's father have a birth defect or genetic condition such as a baby born with an open spine (spina bifida), a heart defect, or Down syndrome?

Yes   No   6.   Does anyone in your family or anyone in the baby's father's family have a birth defect or condition that has been diagnosed as genetic or inherited, such as open spine (spina bifida), a heart defect, or Down syndrome?

Yes   No   7.   Where your ancestors came from may sometimes give us important information about the health of your baby. Are you or the baby's father from any of the following ethnic/racial groups: Jewish, African American, Asian, Mediterranean (Greek, Italian)?

Yes   No   8.   Have you or the baby's father ever been screened to see if you are carriers of the gene for any of the following: Tay-Sachs, sickle cell, thalassemia?

Sometimes, the unborn baby can be exposed to outside factors that can cause birth defects. The next 8 questions will give us important information about possible exposure to the baby.

Yes   No   9.   Have you had any x-rays during this pregnancy?

Yes   No   10. Have you had any alcohol during this pregnancy?

11. Prior to your pregnancy, how often did you drink alcoholic beverages?
☐ Every day   ☐ Less than once a month
☐ At least once a week, not daily   ☐ I do not drink alcoholic beverages.
☐ At least once a month, not weekly

12. Prior to your pregnancy, about how many alcoholic beverages did you usually have per occasion? (1 = one can of beer, one wine cooler, one glass of wine, or one shot of liquor.)
☐ 3 or more
☐ 1 to 2
☐ I do not drink alcoholic beverages.

PRENATAL HISTORY QUESTIONNAIRE - 2

Yes   No   13.   Have you taken any over-the-counter, prescription, or "street" drugs during this pregnancy? If yes, list drugs.

_____

_____

Yes   No   14.   Have you ever sought and/or received treatment for alcohol or drug problems? If yes, how long ago?_____

Yes   No   15.   Do you think you are at increased risk for having a baby with a birth defect or genetic disorder?

Yes   No   16.   At any time during the first 2 months of your pregnancy, have you had a rash or a fever of 103° F or greater?

A test for HIV is strongly recommended for all pregnant women, regardless of your responses to the next questions. The test is voluntary. There are two reasons to be tested: [1] New medications are available to reduce the chance of an infected mother passing HIV to her baby; and [2] most women do not know if they are infected with HIV until late in the disease. Sometimes other infections can put you and your baby at risk. The following questions will help your health care provider determine other areas for counseling and evaluation.

Yes   No   Unsure   17.   Have you or your sexual partners ever had a sexually transmitted infection (STI or VD) such as chlamydia, gonorrhea, syphilis, or herpes?

Yes   No   Unsure   18.   Have you ever had a serious pelvic infection or pelvic inflammatory disease (PID)?

Yes   No   Unsure   19.   Do you think any of your male sexual partners have ever had sex with other men?

Yes   No   Unsure   20.   Have you or your sexual partners ever used IV street drugs?

Yes   No   Unsure   21.   Have you had sex with two or more partners in the last 12 months?

Yes   No   Unsure   22.   Do you think any of your sexual partners may have HIV or AIDS?

Yes   No   Unsure   23.   Have you or your sexual partners ever had a blood transfusion?

How safe you feel in your daily living gives us important information about risks to you and your baby. Please answer these questions as well as you can. All answers will remain private.

        24.   Do you feel safe....

Yes   No   -   in your personal relationship?
Yes   No   -   within your home?
Yes   No   -   in your own neighborhood?
Yes   No   -   other (specify)_____

Yes   No   25.   Have you ever had your feelings repeatedly hurt, been repeatedly put down, or experienced other kinds of hurting?

Yes   No   26.   Are you being or have you ever been hit, slapped, kicked, pushed, or otherwise physically hurt? If yes, by whom?

☐ Husband   ☐ Family member
☐ Ex-husband   ☐ Stranger
☐ Partner   ☐ Other (specify)_____

Yes   No   27.   Are you experiencing or have you ever experienced uncomfortable touching or forced sexual contact? If yes, by whom?

☐ Husband   ☐ Family member
☐ Ex-husband   ☐ Stranger
☐ Partner   ☐ Other (specify)_____

RM/603   REV 6/97

PRENATAL RECORD

DATE	AGE	RACE	RELIGION	OCCUPATION	YRS. ED.	MARITAL STATUS	FATHER OF BABY	FATHER'S WORK PHONE

PHONE-HOME	PHONE-WORK	ADDRESS	REFERRAL-SOURCE	MOTHER'S PRIMARY CARE PROVIDER

GYNECOLOGICAL HISTORY / MEDICAL HISTORY - CONTINUED

GYNECOLOGICAL HISTORY		MEDICAL HISTORY - CONTINUED	
MENARCHE ___ YRS	INTERVAL ___ ☐ REGULAR ☐ IRREGULAR / DURATION ___ DAYS	CARDIOVASCULAR	
		RESPIRATORY/TB	
✔ IF NEGATIVE-DESCRIBE POSITIVE HISTORY		GI	
PAP HISTORY		GU	
INFERTILITY		METABOLIC	
GYN DISORDER		NEURO	
GYN SURGERY		PSYCH-EMOTIONAL	
DES EXPOSURE		HEPATITIS	
PRIOR CONTRACEPTION		MUSCULOSKELETAL	
BCP W/IN 90 DAYS CONCEP		SKIN DISORDERS	
BREASTS		OTHER DISEASE/DX	
OTHER GYN HX		OPERATIONS	
GONORRHEA		TRANSFUSIONS	
SYPHILIS		ALLERGIES	
CHLAMYDIA		FAMILY HISTORY - NOTE IF FATHER OF BABY	
HERPES-SELF/PARTNER		DIABETES	
OTHER STI/HIV		HYPERTENSION	
MEDICAL HISTORY		TWINS	
✔ IF NEGATIVE-DESCRIBE POSITIVE HISTORY		CONGENITAL ANOM	
HEENT		OTHER FAMILY HX	

PREVIOUS PREGNANCIES

NO.	DATE	LENGTH (WKS)	LABOR (HRS)	TYPE DELIVERY	ANES.	SEX	WEIGHT	WHERE DELIVERED	COMPLICATIONS-AP, IP, PP, NEONATAL	OUTCOME/ NAME

PRESENT PREGNANCY HISTORY / PHYSICAL EXAMINATION

PRESENT PREGNANCY HISTORY		PHYSICAL EXAMINATION	DATE
LMP ___ ☐ NORM ☐ ABNORM	LNMP ___ / EDC ___ +PG TEST TYPE DATE	✔ IF NEGATIVE-DESCRIBE POSITIVE FINDINGS	
PLANNED PREGNANCY/OK?	FATHER SUPPORTIVE?	HEIGHT	
		WEIGHT	
✔ IF NEGATIVE-DESCRIBE POSITIVE HISTORY		B.P.	
NAUSEA/VOMITING		HEENT	
BLEEDING		NECK	
URINARY SX		LUNGS	
VAGINAL DISCHARGE		BREASTS	
INFECTION		HEART	
FEVER/RASH		ABDOMEN	
TOBACCO/SMOKING		NEURO	
ETOH		EXTREMITIES/SKIN	
PHYSICAL/SEXUAL ABUSE		PELVIC EXAMINATION	DATE
		EXT. GENITALIA	
PATIENT NO.		VAGINA/CERVIX	
		UTERUS-SIZE	
		PELVIS	
PATIENT NAME		ADNEXA	
		BONY PELVIS/ADEQUATE?	
		HEMORRHOIDS	
D.O.B.		PROVIDER SIGNATURE	

FIRST TRIMESTER			DATE	PROBLEMS AND RISK FACTORS
	DATE	WEEKS	EDC/RANGE		
LMP					
LNMP					
OVU/CONCEP					
FIRST EXAM					
+ HCG URINE					
+ HCG SERUM					
FHT DOPPLER					
FHT FETOSCOPE					
FM					
ULTRASOUND					
ULTRASOUND					
ULTRASOUND					

ANTICIPATORY GUIDANCE

FIRST TRIMESTER	SECOND TRIMESTER	THIRD TRIMESTER
CLINIC PROCEDURES/OUTLINE PRENATAL CARE HIV COUNSELING/TESTING NUTRITION VITAMINS/MINERALS DENTAL/VISION CARE WEIGHT GAIN SEAT BELTS EXERCISE PRENATAL DIAGNOSIS HAZARDS: SMOKING, ETOH, DRUGS, OVERHEATING, CATS, 　　　　　RAW MEAT, UNPASTEURIZED MILK DISCOMFORTS/RELIEF MEASURES WARNING SIGNS: BLEEDING, CRAMPS, ABDOMINAL 　　　　　PAINS, DYSURIA, ETC. BROCHURES	FETAL DEVELOPMENT/QUICKENING FAMILY/FATHER/SIBLINGS HOSPITAL PRE-ADMISSION/TOUR? FEEDING PLANS (BREAST/BOTTLE) EXERCISES/BODY MECHANICS WARNING SIGNS: SROM, BLEEDING, PRE-TERM LABOR BABY'S CARE PROVIDER _____ 　　　　　NEWBORN CARE/ROOMING-IN 　　　　　CIRCUMCISION BROCHURES PRENATAL CLASSES SUPPORT PERSON _____ BIRTH PLANS/OPTIONS SEXUALITY	DISCOMFORTS/RELIEF MEASURES WARNING SIGNS FETAL ACTIVITY MONITORING LABOR SIGNS: WHEN AND HOW TO CALL TRAVEL RESTRICTIONS LABOR & DELIVERY ROUTINE ELECTRONIC FETAL MONITORING ANESTHESIA/ANALGESIA EPISIOTOMY/PERINEAL INTEGRITY LABOR & DELIVERY COMPLICATIONS/OPERATIVE DELIVERY BREAST CARE CAR SEAT DISCUSS POST-TERM MANAGEMENT EARLY DISCHARGE/HELP AT HOME

DATE	MEDICATIONS	POSTPARTUM CONTRACEPTIVE PLANS	
	RHOGAM	☐ ORAL CONTRACEPTION	☐ LONG-ACTING CONTRACEPTION
		☐ STERILIZATION - DATE TUBAL FORM SIGNED _____	
		☐ BARRIER	☐ OTHER
DRUG ALLERGIES/REACTIONS　☐ NKA			
PATIENT NAME			

LABORATORY DATA

TYPE RH		RUBELLA	SEROLOGY	HBsAg	HIV	URINE			DIABETIC SCREEN _____ @ _____ WKS	SICKLE PREP	PPD/TINE

ANTIBODY SCREEN _____ @ _____ WKS _____ @ _____ WKS	HCT _____ @ _____ WKS _____ @ _____ WKS	HSV SEROLOGY I _____ II _____ MSAFP / MOM PAP DATE	CERVICAL CULTURES DATE CHLAMYDIA GC HSV STREP	GTT @ _____ WKS FBS 1 HR _____ 2 HR _____ 3 HR _____	OTHER COPY SENT _____ COPY SENT _____

EDC	REVISED EDC	REVISED EDC	AGE	GRAVIDA	PARA		ABORTIONS			DEATHS		LIVING CHILDREN
					TERM	PRETERM	SPONT	ELEC	ECTOPIC	FETAL	NEONATAL	

WEIGHT AND FUNDAL HEIGHT GRAPH

DATE																								
WEEKS GESTATION	6	8	10	12	14	16	18	20	22	24	26	28	30	32	33	34	35	36	37	38	39	40	41	42	43

CM
40
35
30
25
20

+ 50 #   50 #
+ 40 #   40 #
+ 30 #   30 #
+ 20 #   20 #
+ 10 #   10 #

FUNDAL HEIGHT

WEIGHT

PRENATAL VISITS

WEIGHT NON PG _____																								
BLOOD PRESSURE																								
BLOOD PRESSURE RE-CHECK																								
URINE PROTEIN/ GLUCOSE																								
FHR D-DOPPLER F-FETOSCOPE																								
PRESENTATION																								
ESTIMATE UTERINE SIZE																								
FETAL ACTIVITY																								

WEEKS GESTATION	6	8	10	12	14	16	18	20	22	24	26	28	30	32	33	34	35	36	37	38	39	40	41	42	43
FUTURE PARAMETERS TO CHECK						M S A F P OR TRIPLE SCREEN				HCT DIABETIC SCREEN RhNEG - ANTIBODY SCREEN ? RHOGAM												FETAL SURVEILLANCE			
SEE NOTE (✔)																								
RETURN WEEKS																								
INITIALS																								

PATIENT NO.   HOSPITAL

PATIENT NAME

D.O.B.

RISK FACTOR GUIDELINES	PROGRESS NOTES
PATIENT PROFILE	
AGE > 34 OR PREGNANCY WITHIN 2 YEARS OF MENARCHE	
OCCUPATION AND AVOCATION	
DRUG ABUSE OR ADDICTION	
ALCOHOL	
SMOKING	
COCAINE	
MARIJUANA	
NARCOTICS	
SEDATIVES/HYPNOTICS	
SALICYLATES AND OTHER PGSI'S	
OTHER	
LOW SOCIO-ECONOMIC STATUS	
WELFARE	
EDUCATION < 9TH GRADE	
CROWDED LIVING CONDITIONS	
OTHER	
BODY HABITUS	
SMALL STATURE (< 5 FEET TALL)	
OBESE (> 50# OVER IDEAL WEIGHT FOR HEIGHT)	
UNDERWEIGHT (> 20# UNDER IDEAL WEIGHT FOR HEIGHT)	
MATERNAL BIRTHWEIGHT (LOW BIRTHWEIGHT OR LARGE FOR DATES)	
PARTNER	
MEDICAL OR SURGICAL DISORDERS	
DRUG, SMOKING OR ALCOHOL ABUSE	
OCCUPATION, AVOCATION, HOBBIES	
STI'S (HERPES, URETHRITIS)	
HIV RISK FACTORS	
GYNECOLOGICAL HISTORY	
UTERINE AND CERVICAL ABNORMALITIES	
PAST UTERINE SURGERY (NON-CESAREAN)	
UTERINE ANOMALIES (CONGENITAL ANOMALIES, DES STIGMATA, MYOMATA)	
CERVICAL LACERATIONS OR CONIZATIONS	
MENSTRUAL HISTORY AND GESTATIONAL DATING	
IRREGULAR MENSES OR OLIGOMENORRHEA	
ORAL CONTRACEPTIVE USE PRIOR TO CONCEPTION	
MEDICAL HISTORY	
ANEMIA (HGB < 9.5 OR HCT < 30)	
HEART DISEASE (SYMPTOMATIC OR ASYMPTOMATIC)	
THROMBOEMBOLISM (DURING PREVIOUS PREGNANCY OR PRIOR TO CURRENT PREGNANCY)	
ANTICOAGULANT USE	
CHRONIC HYPERTENSION (BP > 140/90 AT FIRST PRENATAL VISIT)	
ASTHMA OR OTHER CHRONIC LUNG DISEASE	
SEIZURE DISORDER (WITH OR WITHOUT ANTICONVULSANT USE)	
DIABETES MELLITUS (GESTATIONAL OR PREGESTATIONAL)	
HEPATITIS	
HIV RISK FACTORS	
CHRONIC RENAL DISEASE (BUN > 20, CREATININE > 1.2 AT FIRST PRENATAL VISIT)	
PYELONEPHRITIS	
OBSTETRICAL FACTORS	
PARITY	
PRIMIGRAVIDA	
GRAND MULTIPARA (> 4)	
PAST PREGNANCIES	
HABITUAL ABORTION (≥ 3)	
PREMATURE BIRTH (< 37 WEEKS)	
PREMATURE RUPTURE OF MEMBRANES	
LOW BIRTH WEIGHT INFANT (BIRTHWEIGHT < 10TH PERCENTILE FOR DATES)	
LARGE FOR DATES INFANT (BIRTHWEIGHT > 90TH PERCENTILE FOR DATES)	
FETAL OR NEONATAL DEATH	
CONGENITAL ANOMALIES	
SURVIVING NEUROLOGICALLY IMPAIRED INFANT	
CERVICAL INCOMPETENCY	
MIDFORCEP OR DIFFICULT DELIVERY (E.G., SHOULDER DYSTOCIA)	
ABNORMAL LABOR (ARREST OR PROTRACTION DISORDER OF FIRST OR SECOND STAGE)	
ANTEPARTUM HEMORRHAGE (PLACENTAL ABRUPTION, PLACENTA PREVIA)	
BLEEDING PRIOR TO 20 WEEKS	
RH ISOIMMUNIZATION	
PREGNANCY INDUCED HYPERTENSION	
CESAREAN DELIVERY (LOW TRANSVERSE, LOW VERTICAL, CLASSIC, UNKNOWN)	
INTERVAL FROM LAST DELIVERY < 12 MONTHS	
ANESTHESIA INTOLERANCE OR REACTIONS	
PRESENT PREGNANCY	
EMOTIONAL STRESS	
POOR COMPLIANCE	
LATE REGISTRATION FOR CARE	
UNCERTAIN DATES	
FAILURE TO GAIN WEIGHT (< 1/2 # PER WEEK AFTER 12 WEEKS)	
EXCESSIVE WEIGHT GAIN (> 2 # PER WEEK AFTER 12 WEEKS)	
BLEEDING PRIOR TO 20 WEEKS	
LACK OF PREGNANCY NAUSEA AND VOMITING (MORNING SICKNESS)	
PLACENTAL ABRUPTION	
PLACENTA PREVIA	
OTHER VAGINAL BLEEDING	
PREMATURE RUPTURE OF MEMBRANES	
POLYHYDRAMNIOS OR OLIGOHYDRAMNIOS	
THREATENED PREMATURE LABOR	
PATIENT NAME	

RM 612 REV 5/97

Functional Assessment of the Older Adult

PURPOSE

This chapter describes the functional assessment of the older adult using a systems perspective, including the normal changes of aging and ongoing chronic geriatric syndromes. A number of tools that may be used as part of the functional assessment of the older adult are described.

READING ASSIGNMENT

Jarvis: *Physical Examination and Health Assessment,* 6th ed., Chapter 30, pp. 829-846.

MEDIA ASSIGNMENT

Jarvis: *Physical Examination and Health Assessment* DVD Series: Head-to-Toe Examination of the Older Adult.

GLOSSARY

Study the following terms after completing the reading assignment. You should be able to cover the definition on the right and define the term out loud.

Activities of daily living . . . . . . tasks that are necessary for self-care, such as eating/feeding, bathing, grooming, toileting, walking, and transferring

**Advanced activities of
daily living** . . . . activities that an older adult performs as a family member or as a member of society or community, including occupational and recreational activities

Caregiver assessment . . . . assessment of the health and well-being of an individual's caregiver

Caregiver burden . . . . the perceived strain by the person who cares for an elderly, chronically ill, or disabled person

Domains of cognition . . . . domains included in mental status assessments such as attention, memory, orientation, language, visuospatial skills, and higher cognitive functions

Environmental assessment . . . . assessment of an individual's home environment and community system, including hazards in the home

Functional ability . . . . the ability of a person to perform activities necessary to live in modern society; may include driving, using the telephone, or performing personal tasks such as bathing and toileting

Functional assessment . . . . a systematic assessment that includes assessment of an individual's activities of daily living, instrumental activities of daily living, and mobility

Functional status . . . . a person's actual performance of activities and tasks associated with current life roles (as defined by Richmond et al., 2004)

Instrumental activities of
daily living . . . . functional abilities necessary for independent community living, such as shopping, meal preparation, housekeeping, laundry, managing finances, taking medications, and using transportation

Katz Index of Independence
in Activities of Daily Living . . . an instrument that is used to measure physical function in older adults and the chronically ill

Lawton Instrumental
Activities of Daily Living . . . . . an instrument that is used to measure an individual's ability to perform instrumental activities of daily living; it may assist in assessing one's ability to live independently

Physical performance
measures . . . . tests that measure balance, gait, motor coordination, and endurance

Social domain . . . . the domain that focuses on an individual's relationships within family, social groups, and the community

Social networks . . . . informal supports that are accessed by older adults, such as family members and close friends, neighbors, church societies, neighborhood groups, and senior centers

Spiritual assessment . . . . assessment of an individual's spiritual health

STUDY GUIDE

After completing the reading and media assignment, you should be able to answer the following questions in the spaces provided.

1. Explain the differences between functional ability and functional status.

2. Differentiate the following, and provide at least 3 examples of each:

   a. Activities of daily living (ADLs)

   b. Instrumental activities of daily living (IADLs)

   c. Advanced activities of daily living

3. Describe at least 2 instruments that may be used to assess the following:

   a. ADLs

   b. IADLs

   c. Physical performance

4. What are the disadvantages of self-answered ADL and IADL instruments?

5. What are the advantages and disadvantages of instruments that measure physical performance?

6. Discuss at least 2 disorders that may alter an older adult's cognition.

7. What are some indications of possible caregiver burnout?

8. Describe a method of assessing an older adult for depression.

9. Describe 3 contexts of care of an older adult.

10. How would functional assessment differ in the above 3 contexts of care?

11. How does (list 4) driving cessation negatively impact the older adult?

12. Define an environmental assessment and list at least 4 common environmental hazards that may be found in an individual's home.

13. Discuss the best approach when performing a spiritual assessment.

14. Describe special considerations that may affect the assessment of an older adult's functional status.

15. State the priority when assessing an older adult who is in pain.

16. Describe 4 nonpharmacologic interventions to improve sleep in the hospital.

ADDITIONAL LEARNING ACTIVITIES

1. Accompany a nurse practitioner who specializes in the care of older adults as he or she makes rounds in the hospital setting or a long-term care facility.

2. In a clinical setting that focuses on older adults (e.g., a geriatric or psychiatric unit, a daytime geriatric psychiatric program, or a senior citizen center), observe a nurse, occupational therapist, or social worker perform various assessments of older adults.

REVIEW QUESTIONS

This test is for you to check your own mastery of the content. Answers are provided in Appendix A.

1. An appropriate tool to assess an individual's instrumental activities of daily living would be a tool by:

   a. Katz.
   b. Lawton.
   c. Tinetti.
   d. Norbeck.

2. Which of the following statements is true regarding an individual's functional status?

   a. Functional status refers to one's ability to care for another person.
   b. An older adult's functional status is usually static over time.
   c. An older adult's functional status may vary from independence to disability.
   d. Dementia is an example of functional status.

3. An older person is experiencing an acute change in cognition. The nurse recognizes that this disorder is:

   a. Alzheimer dementia.
   b. attention deficit disorder.
   c. depression.
   d. delirium.

4. Assessment of the social domain includes:

   a. family relationships.
   b. the ability to cook meals.
   c. the ability to balance the checkbook and pay bills.
   d. hazards found in the home.

5. The nurse will use which technique when assessing an older individual who has cognitive impairment?

   a. asking open-ended questions
   b. completing the entire assessment in one session
   c. asking the family members for information instead of the older individual
   d. asking simple questions that have "yes" or "no" answers.

6. An older person needs to be assessed before going home as to whether he or she is able to go outside alone safely. The nurse will suggest which test for this assessment?

   a. Up and Go Test
   b. Performance of Activities of Daily Living test
   c. Older Americans Resources and Services Multidimensional Functional Assessment Questionnaire
   d. Lawton IADL instrument

7. The nurse is assessing an older adult who has had surgery for a fractured hip and a history of dementia. The nurse should keep in mind that older adults with cognitive impairment:

   a. experience less pain.
   b. can provide a self-report of pain.
   c. cannot be relied on to self-report pain.
   d. will not express pain sensations.

8. An appropriate use for the Caregiver Strain Index would be which situation?

   a. a daughter who is taking her elderly father home to live with her
   b. an older patient who lives alone
   c. a wife who has cared for her husband for the past 4 years at home
   d. a son whose parents live in an assisted living facility

9. Which of the following is an example of a formal social support network for the aging adult?

   a. a neighbor who drops by with newspapers and magazines on a regular basis
   b. the area church that offers a weekly activity and luncheon for seniors in the neighborhood
   c. the home health care agency that provides weekly blood pressure screenings at the church luncheon
   d. the senior citizen chess club whose members hold classes at the local Boys' Club

10. When completing a spiritual assessment, the examiner should:

    a. use "yes" and "no" questions as the foundation for future dialogue.
    b. use open-ended questions to help the patient understand potential coping mechanisms.
    c. try to complete this assessment as soon as possible after meeting the patient.
    d. wait until a member of the clergy can be involved in the assessment.

SKILLS LABORATORY/CLINICAL SETTING

You are now ready for the clinical component of functional assessment of the older adult. The purpose of the clinical component is to practice portions of a functional assessment either in a clinical setting with older adults (e.g., a geriatric inpatient unit or an assisted living facility) or in the home of an older adult (e.g., a neighbor or family member). In addition, the following should be achieved.

Clinical Objectives

1. Using the Katz Activities of Daily Living instrument, assess the ADLs of an older individual.

2. Assess the safety of the environment of an older person by using the Home Safety Checklist.

Instructions

Katz ADL:
Review the questions on the assessment form. In a clinical setting, such as a long-term care facility or a hospital setting, use the Katz ADL form to assess at least three older individuals. Compare the results of the three assessments. Did you identify any areas of dependence? Did you actually observe the areas, or did the older adult self-report?

Home Safety Checklist:
Review the questions on the checklist, and then practice the assessment in your own home. Did you identify any areas of concern? After practicing at your home, perform this assessment in the home of an older adult, such as a neighbor or a family member. Review the results, and provide suggestions for improving safety as indicated by the assessment.

National Safety Council Home Safety Checklist

Make your home a safer place. Use this checklist to evaluate home hazards.

Outside the house:

Uneven ground? Level problem areas or mark them to prevent a fall.

Do you have ice-melt, salt, or sand for icy driveways, sidewalks, and porches?

Are power tools and hazardous substances like weed killers, fertilizers, or grease-removing solvents locked inside a cabinet, out of children's reach?

Are flammable materials, such as gasoline or oil-soaked rags, in appropriate containers?

Do you keep the garage door down and locked at all times?

Is the automatic reverse mechanism on the garage door working properly? Test it monthly!

If you have a swimming pool, does it have a locked barrier to keep kids out when no adults are around to supervise them?

Inside the house:

When was the last time you tested your smoke alarms? Changed the batteries?

Do you have a fire escape route for your family?

Do you notice any frayed wires, wires under carpets, loose plugs, or gas smells around pipes or appliances?

Do your throw rugs have nonskid padding?

Do your staircases have handrails and slip-resistant floor coverings?

Is there a bath mat near the bathtub or shower?

Are household cleaning products and medications kept out of children's reach? Do they have childproof caps?

Do you have a carbon monoxide detector?

Is the number of your local poison control center posted near every phone?

From *A Year 2000 Home Safety Checklist: Family Safety & Health*, National Safety Council, 2000; *Your Home Safety Checklist*, National Safety Council, 2002; *There's No Place Like Home*, National Safety Council, 2003.

Katz Activities of Daily Living		
Activities Points (1 or 0)	**Independence** (1 point) NO supervision, direction, or personal assistance	**Dependence** (0 points) WITH supervision, direction, personal assistance, or total care
Bathing Points _____	(1 Point) Bathes self completely or needs help in bathing only a single part of the body such as the back, genital area, or disabled extremity	(0 Points) Needs help with bathing more than one part of the body or getting in or out of the tub or shower. Requires total bathing
Dressing Points _____	(1 Point) Gets clothes from closet and drawers and puts on clothes and outer garments complete with fasteners. May have help tying shoes	(0 Points) Needs help with dressing self or needs to be completely dressed
Toileting Points _____	(1 Point) Gets to toilet, gets on and off, arranges clothes, cleans genital area without help	(0 Points) Needs help transferring to the toilet, cleaning self, or using bedpan or commode
Transferring Points _____	(1 Point) Moves in and out of bed or chair unassisted. Mechanical transferring aids are acceptable	(0 Points) Needs help in moving from bed to chair or requires a complete transfer
Continence Points _____	(1 Point) Exercises complete self-control over urination and defecation	(0 Points) Is partially or totally incontinent of bowel or bladder
Feeding Points _____	(1 Point) Gets food from plate into mouth without help. Preparation of food may be done by another person	(0 Points) Needs partial or total help with feeding or requires parenteral feeding
Total points = _____	6 = High (patient independent)	0 = Low (patient very dependent)

Modified from Gerontological Society of America. Katz S, Down TD, Cash HR, & Grotz RC. (1970). Progress in the development of the index of ADL, *The Gerontologist*, 10, 20-30.

NOTES

NOTES

APPENDIX A

Answers to Review Questions

CHAPTER 1: EVIDENCE-BASED ASSESSMENT

1. a
2. d
3. c
4. b
5. c
6. a
7. a
8. c

CHAPTER 2: CULTURAL COMPETENCE: CULTURAL CARE

1. b
2. c
3. d
4. c
5. c
6. a
7. b
8. d

CHAPTER 3: THE INTERVIEW

1. a
2. a
3. b
4. c
5. d
6. b
7. a
8. d
9. b
10. d
11. b
12. c
13. a
14. b
15. b

CHAPTER 4: THE COMPLETE HEALTH HISTORY

1. d
2. a
3. c
4. b
5. c
6. c
7. a
8. d
9. b
10. d

11. P What brings it on? What were you doing when you first noticed it? What makes it better? Worse?

Q How does it look, feel, sound? How intense/severe is it?

R Where is it? Can you point to the location? Does it spread anywhere?

S How bad is it? (on a scale of 0 to 10)? Is it getting better, worse, staying the same?

T When did it first occur? How long did it last? How often does it occur?

U What do you think this means? Is this significant to you?

12. c

CHAPTER 5: MENTAL STATUS ASSESSMENT

1. d
2. a
3. d
4. c
5. b
6. c
7. b
8. c
9. a
10. b
11. a
12. c

13. i
14. d
15. b
16. g
17. f
18. a
19. e

20. h
21. Patient is dressed and groomed appropriately for season and setting. Posture is erect, with no involuntary body movements. Oriented to time, person, and place.

Recent and remote memory intact. Affect and verbal responses appropriate. Perceptions and thought processes logical and coherent.

CHAPTER 6: SUBSTANCE USE ASSESSMENT

1. d
2. c
3. b

4. a
5. c
6. b

7. b
8. c

CHAPTER 7: DOMESTIC VIOLENCE ASSESSMENT

1. d
2. a
3. b
4. b

5. a
6. e
7. d
8. d

9. b
10. c
11. b

CHAPTER 8: ASSESSMENT TECHNIQUES AND THE CLINICAL SETTING

1. d
2. c
3. b
4. a

5. c
6. d
7. c
8. c

9. d
10. a

CHAPTER 9: GENERAL SURVEY, MEASUREMENT, VITAL SIGNS

1. d
2. c
3. b
4. c
5. c

6. a
7. b
8. b
9. d
10. a

11. d
12. c
13. a

CHAPTER 10: PAIN ASSESSMENT: THE FIFTH VITAL SIGN

1. c
2. b
3. c
4. d
5. d

6. b
7. c
8. b
9. d
10. c

11. d
12. b
13. d
14. d

CHAPTER 11: NUTRITIONAL ASSESSMENT

1. c	7. b	13. d
2. d	8. a	14. c
3. c	9. b	15. d
4. c	10. c	16. b
5. c	11. c	
6. b	12. b	

CHAPTER 12: SKIN, HAIR, AND NAILS

1. b	13. c	25. b
2. d	14. c	26. c
3. a	15. a	27. a
4. d	16. b	28. b
5. b	17. c	29. d
6. d	18. a	30. b
7. c	19. a	31. a
8. c	20. c	32. g
9. a	21. b	33. c
10. c	22. c	34. f
11. d	23. a	35. d
12. c	24. a	36. e

CHAPTER 13: HEAD, FACE, AND NECK, INCLUDING REGIONAL LYMPHATICS

1. d	9. a	17. f
2. c	10. a	18. h
3. b	11. a	19. g
4. a	12. c	20. i
5. d	13. a	21. j
6. d	14. b	22. b
7. c	15. c	23. d
8. d	16. e	24. a

CHAPTER 14: EYES

1. b	12. c	positions and back to the center each time. A normal response is parallel tracking of the object with both eyes.
2. c	13. b	
3. a	14. a	
4. b	15. b	
5. d	16. Instruct the patient to hold the head steady and follow the examiner's finger. The examiner holds the finger 12 inches from the individual and moves it clockwise to the 2, 3, 4, 8, 9, and 10 o'clock	17. a. P—pupils
6. c		b. E—equal
7. a		c. R—round
8. c		d. R—react (to)
9. a		e. L—light (and)
10. c		f. A—accommodation
11. b		18. c

CHAPTER 15: EARS

1. c	7. d	13. a
2. a	8. b	14. d
3. d	9. d	15. c
4. b	10. b	16. b
5. a	11. a	
6. c	12. b	

CHAPTER 16: NOSE, MOUTH, AND THROAT

1. c	6. b	11. a
2. d	7. d	12. c
3. a	8. c	13. a
4. a	9. a	
5. b	10. d	

CHAPTER 17: BREASTS AND REGIONAL LYMPHATICS

1. d	7. c	13. d
2. b	8. c	14. a
3. a	9. b	15. b
4. c	10. d	16. b
5. a	11. c	17. c
6. c	12. b	

CHAPTER 18: THORAX AND LUNGS

1. a	10. d	19. d
2. b	11. b	20. b
3. b	12. c	21. e
4. a	13. a	22. a
5. c	14. c	23. d
6. b	15. a	24. f
7. b	16. e	25. c
8. d	17. a	26. b
9. c	18. c	

CHAPTER 19: HEART AND NECK VESSELS

1. c	6. d	11. a
2. b	7. b	12. b
3. c	8. b	13. c
4. b	9. a	14. c
5. d	10. a	15. b

CHAPTER 11: NUTRITIONAL ASSESSMENT

1. c
2. d
3. c
4. c
5. c
6. b

7. b
8. a
9. b
10. c
11. c
12. b

13. d
14. c
15. d
16. b

CHAPTER 12: SKIN, HAIR, AND NAILS

1. b
2. d
3. a
4. d
5. b
6. d
7. c
8. c
9. a
10. c
11. d
12. c

13. c
14. c
15. a
16. b
17. c
18. a
19. a
20. c
21. b
22. c
23. a
24. a

25. b
26. c
27. a
28. b
29. d
30. b
31. a
32. g
33. c
34. f
35. d
36. e

CHAPTER 13: HEAD, FACE, AND NECK, INCLUDING REGIONAL LYMPHATICS

1. d
2. c
3. b
4. a
5. d
6. d
7. c
8. d

9. a
10. a
11. a
12. c
13. a
14. b
15. c
16. e

17. f
18. h
19. g
20. i
21. j
22. b
23. d
24. a

CHAPTER 14: EYES

1. b
2. c
3. a
4. b
5. d
6. c
7. a
8. c
9. a
10. c
11. b

12. c
13. b
14. a
15. b
16. Instruct the patient to hold the head steady and follow the examiner's finger. The examiner holds the finger 12 inches from the individual and moves it clockwise to the 2, 3, 4, 8, 9, and 10 o'clock

positions and back to the center each time. A normal response is parallel tracking of the object with both eyes.

17. a. P—pupils
    b. E—equal
    c. R—round
    d. R—react (to)
    e. L—light (and)
    f. A—accommodation
18. c

CHAPTER 15: EARS

1. c	7. d	13. a
2. a	8. b	14. d
3. d	9. d	15. c
4. b	10. b	16. b
5. a	11. a	
6. c	12. b	

CHAPTER 16: NOSE, MOUTH, AND THROAT

1. c	6. b	11. a
2. d	7. d	12. c
3. a	8. c	13. a
4. a	9. a	
5. b	10. d	

CHAPTER 17: BREASTS AND REGIONAL LYMPHATICS

1. d	7. c	13. d
2. b	8. c	14. a
3. a	9. b	15. b
4. c	10. d	16. b
5. a	11. c	17. c
6. c	12. b	

CHAPTER 18: THORAX AND LUNGS

1. a	10. d	19. d
2. b	11. b	20. b
3. b	12. c	21. e
4. a	13. a	22. a
5. c	14. c	23. d
6. b	15. a	24. f
7. b	16. e	25. c
8. d	17. a	26. b
9. c	18. c	

CHAPTER 19: HEART AND NECK VESSELS

1. c	6. d	11. a
2. b	7. b	12. b
3. c	8. b	13. c
4. b	9. a	14. c
5. d	10. a	15. b

16. Fill in the following blanks:
S$_1$ is best heard at the __apex__ of the heart, whereas S$_2$ is loudest at the __base__ of the heart. S$_1$ coincides with the pulse in the _carotid artery_ and coincides with the __R__ wave if the patient is on an ECG monitor.

17. e
18. c
19. f
20. a
21. b
22. d
23. Liver to right atrium via inferior vena cava, through tricuspid valve to right ventricle, through the pulmonic valve to the pulmonary artery, picks up oxygen in the lungs, returns to left atrium, to left ventricle via mitral valve, through aortic valve to aorta, and out to the body.

24. The major risk factors for heart disease and stroke are hypertension, smoking, high cholesterol levels, obesity, and diabetes. Physical inactivity, family history of heart disease, and age are other risk factors.

CHAPTER 20: PERIPHERAL VASCULAR SYSTEM AND LYMPHATIC SYSTEM

1. a
2. c
3. c
4. b
5. c
6. d
7. a
8. d
9. b
10. d
11. a
12. c
13. a
14. c
15. b
16. b

CHAPTER 21: ABDOMEN

1. c
2. c
3. a
4. d
5. c
6. a
7. d
8. d
9. d
10. a
11. d
12. a
13. c
14. b
15. d
16. Black, tarry stools indicate the present of occult blood (melena) from bleeding higher in the gastrointestinal tract. The blood has been partially broken down during the digestive process. Black, nontarry stools may be caused by ingesting iron supplements. Red blood in stools occurs with localized bleeding in the lower gastrointestinal tract and around the anus, such as occurs with hemorrhoids.

CHAPTER 22: MUSCULOSKELETAL SYSTEM

1. d
2. b
3. d
4. c
5. d
6. a
7. a
8. c
9. b
10. The musculoskeletal system provides support to the body, enabling it to stand erect and to move. The system protects inner organs, produces red blood cells, and provides for the storage of minerals.
11. c
12. b
13. b
14. e
15. g
16. i
17. d
18. a
19. j
20. m
21. k
22. n
23. l
24. h
25. f
26. c

Jarvis, Carolyn: PHYSICAL EXAMINATION AND HEALTH ASSESSMENT: Sixth Edition, Student Laboratory Manual. Copyright © 2012, 2008, 2004, 2000, 1996 by Saunders, an imprint of Elsevier Inc. All rights reserved.

CHAPTER 23: NEUROLOGIC SYSTEM

1. a	10. d	19. h
2. d	11. b	20. c
3. c	12. c	21. l
4. c	13. b	22. d
5. b	14. d	23. i
6. c	15. f	24. e
7. b	16. b	25. j
8. a	17. g	26. a
9. b	18. k	

CHAPTER 24: MALE GENITOURINARY SYSTEM

1. c
2. c
3. d
4. c
5. c
6. d
7. b
8. a
9. d
10. a

11. a
12. b
13. e
14. Voids clear, amber urine 5 or 6 times a day. No nocturia, dysuria, or hesitancy. No pain or discharge from penis. Sexually active with multiple partners. Uses prophylaxis that is satisfactory for both

partners. No history of sexually transmitted infection. No lesions, inflammation, or discharge from penis noted on examination. Testes descended without masses. No inguinal hernia.
15. d
16. b

CHAPTER 25: ANUS, RECTUM, AND PROSTATE

1. a
2. b
3. c
4. a
5. d
6. c
7. b
8. c

9. a
10. No recent change in bowel habits. One soft, dark brown BM daily. No pain or bleeding. No medications. Diet includes 4 servings of fruits and vegetables daily. No hemorrhoids or rectal

lesions noted. Sphincter tone good. No masses or tenderness on palpation. No masses, tenderness, or enlargement of prostate. Stool is Hematest negative.
11. c
12. a

CHAPTER 26: FEMALE GENITOURINARY SYSTEM

1. d
2. a
3. d
4. c
5. c
6. d
7. d
8. b
9. c

10. b
11. b
12. a
13. a
14. Menarche at age 14, cycle 28 to 32 days of 4 to 5 days' duration. Flow moderate with no dysmenorrhea. Gravida 0/Para 0/Ab 0. Has

annual gynecologic exam. No urinary problems, no vaginal discharge. Uses barrier method of birth control. Method satisfactory to self and partner.
15. b
16. b

CHAPTER 29: THE PREGNANT WOMAN

1. c
2. a
3. c
4. a
5. c
6. c
7. b
8. e
9. f
10. f
11. d
12. b
13. c
14. d

15. f
16. Possible answers include:
   a. Fundal height small for dates. Possible causes: inaccurate dates, premature labor, intrauterine growth restriction, fetal position
   b. Fundal height larger for dates. Possible causes: inaccurate dates, hydatidiform mole, multiple fetuses, polyhydramnios, fetal macrosomia
   c. Vaginal bleeding. Possible causes: blighted ovum, friable cervix, ectopic pregnancy, perigestational hemorrhage, cervical lesions, threatened miscarriage, placenta previa, abruptio placentae, uterine rupture

CHAPTER 30: FUNCTIONAL ASSESSMENT OF THE OLDER ADULT

1. b
2. c
3. d
4. a

5. d
6. a
7. b
8. c

9. c
10. b

APPENDIX B

Summary of Infant Growth and Development

Age (months)	Physical Competency	Intellectual Competency	Emotional-Social Competency
1 to 2	Holds head in alignment when prone; Moro reflex to loud sound; follows objects; smiles.	Reflex activity; vowel sounds produced.	Gratification through sucking and basic needs being promptly met; smiles at people.
2 to 4	Turns back to side; raises head and chest 45-90 degrees off bed and supports weight on arms; reaches for objects; follows object through midline; drools; begins to localize sounds; prefers configuration of face.	Reproduces behavior initially achieved by random activity; imitates behavior previously done. Visually studies objects; locates sounds; makes cooing sounds; does not look for objects removed from presence.	Social responsiveness; awareness of those who are not primary caregiver; smiles in response to familiar face.
4 to 6	Birth weight doubled; teeth eruption may begin; sits with stable head and back control; rolls from abdomen to back; picks up object with palmar grasp.	Some intentional actions; some sense of object permanence, looks on same path for vanished object; recognizes partially hidden objects; more systematic in imitative behavior; babbles.	Prefers primary caregiver; sucking needs decrease; laughs in pleasure.
6 to 8	Turns back to stomach; sits alone; crawls; transfers objects hand to hand; turns to sound behind.	Continued development as in 4 to 6 months.	Differentiated response to nonprimary caregivers; evidence of "stranger" or "separation" anxiety.
8 to 10	Creeps; pulls to stand; pincer grasp.	Actions more goal directed; able to solve simple problems by using previously mastered responses. Actively searches for an object that disappears.	Attachment process complete.
10 to 12	Birth weight tripled; cruises; stands by self; may use spoon.	Begins to imitate behavior done before by others but not by self. Understands words being said; may say 1 to 4 words. Intentionality is present.	Begins to explore and separate briefly from parent.

Age (months)	Nutrition	Play	Safety
1 to 2	Breastfed or fortified formula.	Variety of positions. Caregiver should hold and talk to infant. Large, brightly colored objects.	Car carrier; proper use of infant seat.
2 to 4	As for 1 to 2 months.	Talk to and hold. Musical toys; rattle, mobile. Variety of objects of different color, size, and texture; mirror, crib toys, variety of settings.	Do not leave unattended on couch, bed, etc. Remove any small objects that infant could choke on.
4 to 6	Introduction of solids; initial store of iron depletion.	Talk and hold. Provide open space to move and objects to grasp.	Keep environment free of safety hazards; check toys for sharp edges and small pieces that might break.
6 to 8	As for 4 to 6 months.	Provide place to explore. Stack toys, blocks; nursery rhymes.	Check infant's expanding environment for hazards.

Summary of Infant Growth and Development—cont'd

Age (months)	Nutrition	Play	Safety
8 to 10	As for 4 to 6 months.	Games: hide-and-seek, peek-a-boo, pat-a-cake, looking at pictures in a book.	Keep: electrical outlets plugged, cords out of reach, stairs blocked, coffee and end tables cleared of hazards. Do not leave alone in bathtub. Keep poisons out of reach and locked up. Continue use of safety seat in car.
10 to 12	More solids than liquids; increasing use of cup; begin to wean.	Increase space; read to infant. Name and point to body parts. Water and sand play; ball.	As for 8 to 10 months.

Modified from Betz, C., Hunsberger, M., & Wright, S. (1994). *Family-centered nursing care of children* (2nd ed., pp. 148-149). Philadelphia: Saunders.

APPENDIX C

Summary of Toddler Growth, Development, and Health Maintenance

Age	Physical Competency	Intellectual Competency	Emotional-social Competency
General: 1 to 3 yrs	Gains 5 kg (11 lbs). Grows 20.3 cm (8 inches). 12 teeth erupt. Nutritional requirements: Energy 100 Kcal/kg/day Fluid 115-125 mL/kg/day Protein 1.8 gm/kg/day Ask care provider about vitamins and minerals.	Learns by exploring and experimenting. Learns by imitating. Progresses from a vocabulary of 3 or 4 words at 12 months to about 900 words at 36 months.	Central crisis: to gain a sense of experimenting autonomy versus doubt and shame. Demonstrates independent behaviors. Exhibits attachment behavior strongly and regularly until third birthday. Fears persist of strange people, objects, and places and of aloneness and being abandoned. Egocentric in play (parallel play). Imitation of parents in household tasks and activities of daily living.
15 months	Legs appear bowed. Walks alone, climbs, slides downstairs backward. Stacks two blocks. Scribbles spontaneously. Grasps spoon but rotates it, holds cup with both hands. Takes off socks and shoes.	Trial-and-error method of learning. Experiments to see what will happen. Says at least three words. Uses expressive jargon.	Shows independence by trying to feed self and helps in undressing.
18 months	Runs but still falls. Walks upstairs with help. Slides downstairs backwards. Stacks three to four blocks. Clumsily throws a ball. Unzips a large zipper. Takes off simple garments.	Begins to maintain a mental image of an absent object. Concept of object permanence fully develops. Has vocabulary of 10 or more words. Holophrastic speech (one word used to communicate whole ideas).	Fears the water. Temper tantrums may begin. Negativism and dawdling predominate. Bedtime rituals begin. Awareness of gender identity begins. Helps with undressing.

Continued

Summary of Toddler Growth, Development, and Health Maintenance—cont'd

Age	Physical Competency	Intellectual Competency	Emotional-social Competency
24 months	Runs quickly and with fewer falls. Pulls toys and walks sideways. Walks downstairs hanging onto a rail (does not alternate feet). Stacks six blocks. Turns pages of a book. Imitates vertical and circular strokes. Uses spoon with little spilling. Can feed self. Puts on simple garments. Can turn door knobs.	Enters into preconceptual phase of preoperational period: Symbolic thinking and symbolic play. Egocentric thinking, imagination, and pretending are common. Has vocabulary of about 300 words. Uses two-word sentences (telegraphic speech). Engages in monologue.	Fears the dark and animals. Temper tantrums may continue. Negativism and dawdling continue. Bedtime rituals continue. Sleep resisted overtly. Usually shows readiness to begin bowel and bladder control. Explores genitalia. Brushes teeth with help. Helps with dressing and undressing.
36 months	Has set of deciduous teeth at about 30 months. Walks downstairs alternating feet. Rides tricycle. Walks with balance and runs well. Stacks eight to ten blocks. Can pour from a pitcher. Feeds self completely. Dresses self almost completely (does not know front from back). Cannot tie shoes.	Preconceptual phase of preoperational period as for 24 months. Uses around 900 words. Constructs complete sentences and uses all parts of speech.	Temper tantrums subside. Negativism and dawdling subside. Bedtime rituals subside. Self-care in feeding, elimination and dressing enhances self-esteem.

Age	Nutrition	Play	Safety
General: 1 to 3 yrs	Milk 16–24 oz. Appetite decreases. Wants to feed self. Has food jags. Never force food; give nutritious snacks. Give iron and vitamin supplementation only if poor intake.	Books at all stages. Needs physical and quiet activities, does not need expensive toys.	Never leave alone in tub. Keep poisons, including detergents and cleaning products, out of reach. Use car seat.
15 months	Vulnerable to iron deficiency anemia. Give table foods except for tough meat and hard vegetables. Wants to feed self.	Stuffed animals, dolls, music toys. Peek-a-boo, hide-and-seek. Water and sand play. Stacking toys. Roll ball on floor. Push toys on floor. Read to toddler.	Keep small items off floor (pins, buttons, clips). Child may choke on hard food. Cords and tablecloths are a danger. Keep electrical outlets plugged and poisons locked away. Risk of kitchen accidents with toddler under foot.
18 months	Negativism may interfere with eating. Encourage self-feeding. Is easily distracted while eating. May play with food. High activity level interferes with eating.	Rocking horse. Nesting toys. Shapesorting cube. Pencil or crayon. Pull toys. Four-wheeled toy ride. Throw ball. Running and chasing games. Roughhousing. Puzzles. Blocks. Hammer and peg board.	Falls: from riding toy, in bathtub, from running too fast. Climbs up to get dangerous objects. Keep dangerous things out of wastebasket.
24 months	Requests certain foods; therefore snacks should be controlled. Imitates eating habits of others. May still play with food and especially with utensils and dish (pouring, stacking).	Clay and Play-Doh. Finger paint. Brush paint. Music player with story book and songs to sing along. Toys to take apart. Toy tea sets. Puppets. Puzzles.	May fall from outdoor large play equipment. Can reach farther than expected (knives, razors, and matches must be kept out of reach).
36 months	Sits in booster seat rather than highchair. Verbal about likes and dislikes.	Likes playing with other children, building toys, drawing and painting, doing puzzles. Imitation household objects for doll play. Nurse and doctor kits. Carpenter kits.	Protect from turning on hot water, falling from tricycle, striking matches.

Modified from Betz, C., Hunsberger, M., & Wright, S. (1994). *Family-centered nursing care of children* (2nd ed., pp. 190-191). Philadelphia: Saunders.

APPENDIX D

Growth, Development, and Health Promotion for Preschoolers

Age (yrs)	Physical Competency	Intellectual Competency	Emotional-Social Competency
General: 3 to 5	Gains 4.5 kg (10 lbs). Grows 15 cm (6 inches). 20 teeth present. Nutritional requirements: Energy: 1250 to 1600 cal/day (or 90 to 100 Kcal/kg/day) Fluid: 100 to 125 mL/kg/day Protein: 30 g/day (or 3 g/kg/day) Iron: 10 mg/day	Becomes increasingly aware of self and others. Vocabulary increases from 900 to 2100 words. Piaget's preoperational/intuitive period.	Freud's phallic stage. Oedipus complex—boy. Electra complex—girl. Erikson's stage of Initiative vs. Guilt.
3	Runs, stops suddenly. Walks backward. Climbs steps. Jumps. Pedals tricycle. Undresses self. Unbuttons front buttons. Feeds self well.	Knows own sex. Sense of humor. Desires to please. Language—900 words. Follows simple direction. Uses plurals. Names figure in picture. Uses adjectives/adverbs.	Shifts between reality and imagination. Bedtime rituals. Negativism decreases. Animism and realism: anything that moves is alive.
4	Runs well, skips clumsily. Hops on one foot. Heel-toe walks. Up and down steps without holding rail. Jumps well. Dresses and undresses. Buttons well, needs help with zippers, bows. Brushes teeth. Bathes self. Draws with some form and meaning.	More aware of others. Uses alibis to excuse behavior. Bossy. Language—1500 words. Talks in sentences. Knows nursery rhymes. Counts to 5. Highly imaginative. Name calling.	Focuses on present. Egocentrism/unable to see the viewpoint of others, unable to understand another's inability to see own viewpoint. Does not comprehend anticipatory explanation. Sexual curiosity. Oedipus complex. Electra complex.
5	Runs skillfully. Jumps 3–4 steps. Jumps rope, hops, skips. Begins dance. Roller skates. Dresses without assistance. Ties shoelaces. Hits nail on head with hammer. Draws person—6 parts. Prints first name.	Aware of cultural differences. Knows name and address. More independent. More sensible/less imaginative. Copies triangle, draws rectangle. Knows four or more colors. Language—2100 words, meaningful sentences. Understands kinship. Counts to 10.	Continues in egocentrism. Fantasy and daydreams. Resolution of Oedipus/Electra complex, girls identify with mother, boys with father. Body image and body boundary especially important in illness. Shows tension in nail-biting, nose-picking, whining, snuffling.

Age (yrs)	Nutrition	Play	Safety
General: 3 to 5	Carbohydrate intake approximately 40 to 50 percent of calories. Good food sources of essential vitamins and minerals. Regular tooth brushing. Parents are seen as examples; if parent won't eat it, child won't.	Reading books is important at all ages. Balance highly physical activities with quiet times. Quiet rest period takes the place of nap time. Provide sturdy play materials.	Never leave alone in bath or swimming pool. Keep poisons in locked cupboard; learn what household things are poisonous. Use car seats and seatbelts. Never leave child alone in car. Remove doors from abandoned refrigerators.

Continued

Growth, Development, and Health Promotion for Preschoolers—cont'd

Age (yrs)	Nutrition	Play	Safety
3	1250 cal/day. Because of increased sex identity and imitation, copies parents at table and will eat what they eat. Different colors and shapes of foods can increase interest.	Participates in simple games. Cooperates, takes turns. Plays with group. Uses scissors, paper. Likes crayons, coloring books. Enjoys being read to and "reading." Plays "dress-up" and "house." Likes fire engines.	Teach safety habits early. Let water out of bathtub; don't stand in tub. Caution against climbing in unsafe areas, onto or under cars, unsafe buildings, drainage pipes. Insist on seatbelts worn at all times in cars.
4	Good nutrition. 1400 cal/day. Nutritious between-meal snacks essential. Emphasis on quality not quantity of food eaten. Mealtime should be enjoyable, not for criticism. As dexterity improves, neatness increases.	Longer attention span with group activities. "Dress-up" with more dramatic play. Draws, pounds, paints. Likes making paper chains, sewing cards. Scrapbooks. Likes being read to, listening to music, and rhythmic play. "Helps" adults.	Teach to stay out of streets, alleys. Continually teach safety; child understands. Teach how to handle scissors. Teach what are poisons and why to avoid. Never allow child to stand in moving car.
5	Good nutrition. 1600 cal/day. Encourage regular tooth brushing. Encourage quiet time before meals. Can learn to cut own meat. Frequent illnesses from increased exposure increase nutritional needs.	Plays with trucks, cars, soldiers, dolls. Likes simple games with letters or numbers. Much gross motor activity: water, mud, snow, leaves, rocks. Matching picture games.	Teach child how to cross streets safely. Teach child not to speak to strangers or get into cars of strangers. Insist on seatbelts. Teach child to swim.

Modified from Betz, C., Hunsberger, M., & Wright, S. (1994). *Family-centered nursing care of children* (2nd ed., pp. 235-236). Philadelphia: Saunders.

APPENDIX E

Competency Development of the School-Age Child

Age (yrs)	Physical Competency	Intellectual Competency	Emotional-Social Competency
General: 6 to 12	Gains an average of 2.5 to 3.2 kg/year (5½ to 7 lbs/year). Overall height gains of 5.5 cm (2 inches) per year; growth occurs in spurts and is mainly in trunk and extremities. Loses deciduous teeth; most of permanent teeth erupt. Progressively more coordinated in both gross and fine motor skills. Caloric needs increase with growth spurts.	Masters concrete operations. Moves from egocentrism; learns he or she is not always right. Learns grammar and expression of emotions and thoughts. Vocabulary increases to 3000 words or more; handles complex sentences.	Central crisis: industry vs. inferiority; wants to do and make things. Progressive sex education needed. Wants to be like friends; competition important. Fears body mutilation, alterations in body image; earlier phobias may recur, nightmares; fears death. Nervous habits common.
6 to 7	Gross motor skill exceeds fine motor coordination. Balance and rhythm are good—runs, skips, jumps, climbs, gallops. Throws and catches ball. Dresses self with little or no help.	Vocabulary of 2500 words. Learning to read and print; beginning concrete concepts of numbers, general classification of items. Knows concepts of right and left; morning, afternoon, and evening; coinage. Intuitive thought process. Verbally aggressive, bossy, opinionated, argumentative. Likes simple games with basic rules.	Boisterous, outgoing, and a know-it-all, whiney; parents should sidestep power struggles, offer choices. Becomes quiet and reflective during 7th year; very sensitive. Can use telephone. Likes to make things: starts many, finishes few. Give some responsibility for household duties.
8 to 10	Myopia may appear. Secondary sex characteristics begin in girls. Hand-eye coordination and fine motor skills well established. Movements are graceful, coordinated. Cares for own physical needs completely. Constantly on move; plays and works hard; enforce balance in rest and activity.	Learning correct grammar and to express feelings in words. Likes books he or she can read alone; will read funny papers, scan newspaper. Enjoys making detailed drawings. Mastering classification, seriation, spatial and temporal, numerical concepts. Uses language as a tool; likes riddles, jokes, chants, word games. Rules guiding force in life now. Very interested in how things work, what and how weather, seasons, etc., are made.	Strong preference for same-sex peers; antagonizes opposite-sex peers. Self-assured and pragmatic at home; questions parental values and ideas. Has a strong sense of humor. Enjoys clubs, group projects, outings, large groups, camp. Modesty about own body increases over time; sex conscious. Works diligently to perfect skills he or she does best. Happy, cooperative, relaxed, and casual in relationships. Increasingly courteous and well-mannered with adults. Gang stage at a peak; secret codes and rituals prevail. Responds better to suggestion than dictatorial approach.
11 to 12	Vital signs approximate adult norms. Growth spurt for girls; inequalities between sexes are increasingly noticeable; boys have greater physical strength. Eruption of permanent teeth complete except for third molars. Secondary sex characteristics begin in boys. Menstruation may begin.	Able to think about social problems and prejudices; sees others' points of view. Enjoys reading mysteries, love stories. Begins playing with abstract ideas. Interested in whys of health measures and understands human reproduction. Very moralistic; religious commitment often made during this time.	Intense team loyalty; boys begin teasing girls and girls flirt with boys for attention; best friend period. Wants unreasonable independence. Rebellious about routine; wide mood swings; needs some time daily for privacy. Very critical of own work. Hero worship prevails. "Facts of life" chats with friends prevail; masturbation increases. Appears under constant tension.
General: 6 to 12	Fluctuations in appetite due to uneven growth pattern and tendency to get involved in activities. Tendency to neglect breakfast owing to rush of getting to school. Though school lunch is provided in most schools, child does not always eat it.	Plays in groups, mostly of same sex; "gang" activities predominate. Books for all ages. Bicycles important. Sports equipment. Cards, board and table games. Most of play is active games requiring little or no equipment.	Enforce continued use of safety belts during car travel. Bicycle safety must be taught and enforced. Teach safety related to hobbies, handicrafts, mechanical equipment.

Continued

Competency Development of the School-Age Child—cont'd

Age (yrs)	Physical Competency	Intellectual Competency	Emotional-Social Competency
6 to 7	Preschool food dislikes persist. Tendency for deficiencies in iron, vitamin A, and riboflavin. 100 mL/kg of water per day. 3 gm/kg protein daily.	Still enjoys dolls, cars, and trucks. Plays well alone but enjoys small groups of both sexes; begins to prefer same sex peer during 7th year. Ready to learn how to ride a bicycle. Prefers imaginary, dramatic play with real costumes. Begins collecting for quantity, not quality. Enjoys active games such as hide-and-seek, tag, jumprope, roller skating, kickball. Ready for lessons in dancing, gymnastics, music. Restrict TV and electronics time to 1-2 hours/day.	Teach and reinforce traffic safety. Still needs adult supervision of play. Teach to avoid strangers, never take anything from strangers. Teach illness prevention and reinforce continued practice of other health habits. Restrict bicycle use to home ground; no traffic areas; teach bicycle safety. Teach the harmful use of drugs, alcohol, smoking. Set a good example.
8 to 10	Needs about 2100 calories/day; nutritious snacks. Tends to be too busy to bother to eat. Tendency for deficiencies in calcium, iron, and thiamine. Problem of obesity may begin now. Good table manners. Able to help with food preparation.	Likes hiking, sports. Enjoys cooking, woodworking, crafts. Enjoys cards and table games. Likes radio and music. Begins qualitative collecting now. Continue restriction on TV and electronics time.	Stress safety with firearms. Keep them out of reach, and allow use only with adult supervision. Know who the child's friends are; parents should still have some control over friend selection. Teach water safety; swimming should be supervised by an adult.
11 to 12	Male needs 2500 calories per day; female needs 2250 (70 cal/kg/day). 75 mL/kg of water per day. 2 gm/kg protein daily.	Enjoys projects and working with hands. Likes to do errands and jobs to earn money. Very involved in sports, dancing, talking on phone. Enjoys all aspects of acting and drama.	Continue monitoring friends; stress bicycle safety on streets and in traffic.

Modified from Betz, C., Hunsberger, M., & Wright, S. (1994). *Family-centered nursing care of children* (2nd ed., pp. 281-282). Philadelphia: Saunders.

APPENDIX F

Characteristics of Adolescents

Early Adolescence (12 to 14 yrs)	Middle Adolescence (15 to 16 yrs)	Late Adolescence (17 to 21 yrs)
Becomes comfortable with own body; egocentric. Difficulty solving problems; thinks in present; cannot use past experience to control behavior; sense of invulnerability—society's rules do not apply to him or her. Struggle between dependent and independent behavior; begins forming peer alliance. Parent-child conflict begins; teen argues but without logic.	"Tries out" adultlike behavior. Begins to solve problems, analyze, and abstract. Established peer group alliance with associated risk-taking behavior. Peak turmoil in child-family relations; able to debate issues and use some logic but not continuously.	Aware of own strengths and limitations; establishes own value system. Able to verbalize conceptually: deals with abstract moral concepts; makes decisions regarding future. Peer group diminishes in importance; may develop first intimate relationship. Turbulence subsides. May move away from home. More adultlike friendship with parents.

From Foster, R., Hunsberger, M., & Anderson, J.J. (1989). *Family-centered nursing care of children* (p. 359). Philadelphia: Saunders.

APPENDIX G

Functional Health Patterns Guide

The following table is a general guide for programs employing a functional health patterns approach to assessment.

Functional Health Patterns	Potential Correlating Chapters in the Text
Health Perception—Health Management	• Chapter 3, The Interview • Chapter 4, The Complete Health History • Chapter 30, Functional Assessment of the Older Adult
Nutritional—Metabolic	• Chapter 11, Nutritional Assessment • Chapter 9, General Survey, Measurement, Vital Signs • Chapter 12, Skin, Hair, and Nails • Chapter 16, Nose, Mouth, and Throat • Chapter 21, Abdomen
Elimination	• Chapter 21, Abdomen • Chapter 24, Male Genitourinary System • Chapter 25, Anus, Rectum, and Prostate • Chapter 26, Female Genitourinary System
Activity—Exercise	• Chapter 18, Thorax and Lungs • Chapter 19, Heart and Neck Vessels • Chapter 20, Peripheral Vascular System and Lymphatic System • Chapter 22, Musculoskeletal System
Sleep—Rest	• Chapter 4, The Complete Health History
Cognitive—Perception	• Chapter 5, Mental Status Assessment • Chapter 10, Pain Assessment: The Fifth Vital Sign • Chapter 13, Head, Face, and Neck, Including Regional Lymphatics • Chapter 14, Eyes • Chapter 15, Ears • Chapter 16, Nose, Mouth, and Throat • Chapter 23, Neurologic System • Chapter 30, Functional Assessment of the Older Adult
Self-Perception—Self-Concept	• Chapter 5, Mental Status Assessment • Chapter 30, Functional Assessment of the Older Adult
Role—Relationship	• Chapter 2, Cultural Competence: Cultural Care • Chapter 7, Domestic Violence Assessment • Chapter 30, Functional Assessment of the Older Adult
Sexuality—Reproductive	• Chapter 17, Breasts and Regional Lymphatics • Chapter 24, Male Genitourinary System • Chapter 26, Female Genitourinary System • Chapter 29, The Pregnant Woman
Coping—Stress Tolerance	• Chapter 30, Functional Assessment of the Older Adult
Value—Belief	• Chapter 2, Cultural Competence: Cultural Care